THE DAY I GOT UP

A Story of Healing, Hope, and the Power of Faith

BY EUNICE NEWTON

All rights reserved under the international and Pan-American copyright conventions.

First published in the United States of America.

All rights reserved. With the exception of brief quotations in a review, no part of this book may be reproduced or transmitted, in any form, or by any means, electronic or mechanical (including photocopying), nor may it be stored in any information storage and retrieval system without written permission from the publisher.

DISCLAIMER

The advice contained in this material might not be suitable for everyone. The author designed the information to present her opinion about the subject matter. The reader must carefully investigate all aspects of any business decision before committing to him or herself. The author obtained the information contained herein from sources she believes to be reliable and from her own personal experience, but she neither implies nor intends any guarantee of accuracy. The author is not in the business of giving legal, accounting, or any other type of professional advice. Should the reader need such advice, he or she must seek services from a competent professional. The author particularly disclaims any liability, loss, or risk taken by individuals who directly or indirectly act on the information contained herein. The author believes the advice presented here is sound, but readers cannot hold her responsible for either the actions they take, or the risk taken by individuals who directly or indirectly act on the information contained herein.

Published by 1BrickPublishing
Printed in the United States
Copyright © 2025 by Eunice Newton
ISBN 979-8-89856-024-9

DEDICATION

To my children— You are my heartbeat, my purpose, and the reason I get up every day. Your love gives me strength, your smiles give me joy, and your belief in me keeps me fighting.

To my cousin— Though you're no longer here in body, your spirit walks with me. This book carries the words you never got to share. I pray it helps others the way your love helped me.

And to every person battling something they didn't ask for—May this book remind you that healing starts the moment you decide to get up.

You are not alone. You are not broken. You are powerful.

—Eunice Newton

DEDICATION REQUEST

Please share this book with anyone who's ever felt broken, battled in silence, or needed a reminder that their story isn't over—and that getting up is the first step toward healing.

TABLE OF CONTENTS

INTRODUCTION: THE VOICE YOU NEED TO HEAR 1
PART I: BEFORE THE STORM 7
    CHAPTER 1: THE DAY I GOT UP 9
    CHAPTER 2: BEFORE THE BREAKDOWN.................15
    CHAPTER 3: SIGNS I CHOSE TO IGNORE.................21
PART II: THE DIAGNOSIS 29
    CHAPTER 4: FIVE DAYS THAT CHANGED MY LIFE 31
    CHAPTER 5: WHAT IS MS? 39
    CHAPTER 6: THE BREAKDOWN........................ 45
PART III: FIGHTING BACK........................ 51
    CHAPTER 7: CLAIMING MY FIGHT, NOT MY ILLNESS... 53
    CHAPTER 8: FAITH AND FAMILY GOT ME UP 59
    CHAPTER 9: THAT SUNDAY MORNING VOICE 67
PART IV: LEARNING TO LIVE AGAIN...............75
    CHAPTER 10: WHAT DOES MS LOOK LIKE?.............. 77
    CHAPTER 11: THIS BODY MAY BE SLOWER, BUT THIS SPIRIT IS FIRE...83
    CHAPTER 12: MY KIDS ARE MY PULSE...................89
PART V: FINDING PURPOSE IN PAIN 97
    CHAPTER 13: FROM PAIN TO PURPOSE 99

CHAPTER 14: THE SUPPORT SYSTEM THAT SAVED ME. .107

CHAPTER 15: LIVE. DON'T CLAIM IT. .115

PART VI: MESSAGES FOR WARRIORS. 123

    CHAPTER 16: YOU CAN GET UP TOO. 125

    CHAPTER 17: TAKE CARE OF YOURSELF 131

    CHAPTER 18: LETTER FROM EUNICE 139

    ACKNOWLEDGMENTS 145

    RESOURCES FOR MS AWARENESS AND SUPPORT 151

    ABOUT THE AUTHOR. 155

INTRODUCTION

THE VOICE YOU NEED TO HEAR

Hey, beautiful.

Yeah, I'm talking to you—the one reading this right now, maybe in your bed at 2 AM because sleep won't come, or sitting in a doctor's waiting room with your heart pounding, or hiding in your car after getting news that changed everything. I'm talking to you, the one who picked up this book because something inside you is fighting, even when everything else feels like it's falling apart.

My name is Eunice Newton, but everybody calls me Tweety. I'm a forty-year-old mother of three from Harlem, New York, and I want you to know something right up front—I didn't write this book because I'm some kind of superhero. I wrote it because I'm human, just like you. I wrote it because five years ago, I thought my life was over. I wrote it because I know what it feels like to wake up in a body that doesn't feel like yours anymore, in a life that doesn't look like what you planned.

I wrote this book because I got up.

And if you're reading this, then somewhere deep inside, you're ready to get up too.

Before we go any further, let me tell you what this book is not. This isn't one of those perfect, pretty stories where everything works out neat and clean. This isn't about some woman who got sick and suddenly became enlightened and grateful for every moment. Nah, that's not me, and that's probably not you either.

This book is about the messy, ugly, beautiful, powerful truth of what it means to fight for your life when life decides to fight you back. This is about crying in hospital beds and getting mad at God and feeling like giving up is the only option that makes sense. But it's also about discovering that you're stronger than you ever imagined, that your support system is bigger than you knew, and that sometimes the worst thing that happens to you can become the thing that saves not just you, but everybody who needs to hear your story.

See, five years ago, I was diagnosed with Multiple Sclerosis. MS. Before that day, I had never even heard those words put together. I was a teaching assistant, always on my feet, always moving, always doing for everybody else. I had my son, my daughters, my man, my community. I was the girl from Harlem everybody knew, the one who didn't sit still, the one who showed up for everyone.

Then one day, my boss noticed me limping. "That's not normal," he said, and sent me to the hospital. Five days later, my entire world had changed. The doctor looked at me with those sympathetic eyes and said, "I'm sorry to let you know this, but you have MS."

I'm like, "What is that? What is MS?"

INTRODUCTION: THE VOICE YOU NEED TO HEAR

"Multiple Sclerosis."

"Okay, like what's the problem? Can this be cured? Can I just take some medicine and call it a day?"

The answer was no. There was no quick fix, no magic pill, no going back to the woman I was before.

For months after that, I wanted to die. I'm not going to sugarcoat it for you because that's not what you need right now. You need the truth. I laid in that bed thinking about ending it all because I couldn't see how I was supposed to live with this new reality. I couldn't see how the woman who never sat still was supposed to navigate the world with a cane, with fatigue, with a body that felt like it was betraying her every single day.

But here's what I learned: your lowest moment isn't your final moment. That place where you can't see any way forward? That's not where your story ends. That's where it gets interesting.

Because one Sunday morning, I heard a voice. Maybe it was God, maybe it was my father who had passed away, maybe it was my own spirit refusing to give up—but I heard it clear as day: "Girl, if you don't get your behind out of this bed, you can do it. You can do it."

And that was the day I got up.

Not just physically, though that was part of it. I got up mentally. Spiritually. Emotionally. I got up and decided that MS might be in my body, but it wasn't going to be my story. I got up and decided that I wasn't going to claim this sickness as my identity. I got up and decided that if I was going through this, then maybe—just maybe—I could help somebody else get up too.

That's why you're holding this book right now.

Maybe you don't have MS. Maybe your battle is depression, or divorce, or loss, or addiction, or trauma, or financial struggle, or raising kids alone, or caring for aging parents, or dealing with racism, or fighting cancer, or recovering from abuse. Maybe your battle doesn't even have a name yet—it's just this weight on your chest that makes every day feel like climbing a mountain.

I don't need to know the details of your struggle to know this: you're stronger than you think you are. You have more fight in you than you realize. And you deserve to live a full, beautiful, powerful life, even—especially—in the middle of whatever storm you're weathering right now.

This book is going to take you through my journey—the ugly parts and the beautiful parts, the moments I wanted to give up and the moments I felt like I could conquer the world. I'm going to tell you about my kids who keep me going, my doctor who became my therapist, my friends who wouldn't let me disappear, and my faith that caught me when I was falling.

But more than that, I'm going to tell you about the moment everything changed. The moment I realized that just because life knocked me down didn't mean I had to stay down. The moment I understood that my circumstances don't define me—my response to them does.

I'm going to tell you what I tell everyone who asks me how I do it: "It's a minor thing. Don't claim it. Live your life."

And I'm going to show you how to do exactly that.

INTRODUCTION: THE VOICE YOU NEED TO HEAR

You picked up this book for a reason. Maybe somebody recommended it, maybe you saw it somewhere and the title spoke to you, maybe you're just desperately looking for somebody, anybody, who understands what you're going through. However you got here, you're here. And that means you're ready.

You're ready to hear that you're not alone. You're ready to hear that what you're going through, as hard as it is, doesn't have to be the end of your story. You're ready to hear that you have permission to feel everything you're feeling and then make a choice about what comes next.

You're ready to get up.

So let's do this together, beautiful. Let's walk through this storm and come out the other side. Let's figure out how to live our lives to the fullest, how to take care of ourselves, how to lean on our people, and how to become the voice that somebody else needs to hear.

Let's turn your mess into your message, your pain into your purpose, your breakdown into your breakthrough.

Let's get up and show the world what resilience looks like when it wears your face.

Are you ready? Because I've been waiting for you.

Let's go.

With love and hope, Eunice "Tweety" Newton

PART I: BEFORE THE STORM

CHAPTER 1

THE DAY I GOT UP

I remember that Sunday morning like it was yesterday. The sunlight was trying to creep through my bedroom curtains, but I had been laying in that bed for days—maybe weeks—just staring at the ceiling. My kids would come check on me, my family would call, but I couldn't move. Not because my body wouldn't let me, though that was part of it. I couldn't move because my spirit was broken.

It had been months since the diagnosis. Months since I heard those two letters that changed my entire world: M.S. Multiple Sclerosis. Months of trying to figure out how to live in a body that felt like it belonged to somebody else, how to be a mother when I could barely take care of myself, how to have hope when the future felt like a question mark, I was too afraid to answer.

The depression had me in a chokehold. I'm not going to lie to you about that. There were days—too many days—when I thought about just not being here anymore. The pain wasn't just physical, though Lord knows my right leg felt like it was on fire, and my balance was so off I had to hold onto walls just to walk across the room. The pain was deeper than that. It was the pain of watching your life change overnight and not knowing if you're strong enough to handle what comes next.

But that Sunday morning, something was different.

I was laying there in my usual spot—same position, same emptiness, same wall of grief surrounding me like a thick blanket I couldn't kick off—when I heard it. Clear as day, loud as thunder, real as the breath in my lungs.

"Girl, if you don't get your behind out of this bed. You can do it. You can do it."

Now, I know some of y'all reading this might think I was losing my mind. Maybe I was. But I heard that voice, and it wasn't my voice. It was stronger than my voice, more sure than my voice. It sounded like my father, who had passed away and was a deacon, a man of God who never let anything keep him down. It sounded like every ancestor who had fought battles I couldn't even imagine so I could be here, laying in this bed, having the luxury of giving up.

"You can do it."

I sat up. I don't know why, but I sat up. For the first time in I don't know how long, I actually sat up in that bed and looked around my room. Really looked around. I saw the pictures of my kids on the dresser—my baby boy who was only eight years old then, my daughter who was about to graduate college, my other daughter who needed her mama to show her what strength looked like. I saw the cards people had sent me, the flowers that had died because I couldn't even take care of plants, the life that was waiting for me to rejoin it.

CHAPTER 1: THE DAY I GOT UP

And something inside me shifted.

It wasn't like the movies where everything suddenly becomes clear and you feel amazing and ready to conquer the world. Nah, it wasn't like that at all. I still felt heavy. I still felt scared. My leg still hurt, and I still didn't know what tomorrow was going to look like or how I was going to navigate this thing called MS.

But I felt something I hadn't felt in months: possibility.

Maybe—just maybe—I could figure this out. Maybe—just maybe—this wasn't the end of my story but the beginning of a different chapter. Maybe—just maybe—I was stronger than I thought I was.

I swung my legs over the side of the bed. That simple movement that used to be automatic now took effort, concentration, courage. But I did it. I put my feet on the floor, and I stood up.

My kid's grandmother called me right then. I swear, it was like she knew. That woman had a sixth sense about her grandbabies, and she always seemed to call right when we needed her most.

"Tweety," she said—that's what everybody calls me, and I used to hate that nickname, but hearing it in her voice that morning felt like love itself. "Are you okay? I'm not used to you being in bed like this. You've been in that bed for days."

She was right. The old me never stayed still. Even as a kid, I was always moving, always doing something, always going somewhere. I couldn't sit still if my life depended on it. And here I was, letting this illness convince me that staying still was my only option.

11

"Something's wrong," she asked. "I'm going to send my sister over to check on you."

After we hung up, I looked at myself in the mirror. Really looked. I saw a woman I barely recognized—hair all over the place, eyes that had lost their spark, shoulders carrying the weight of a diagnosis I was still trying to understand. But I also saw something else. I saw fight. It was buried under all that pain and fear, but it was there.

Her sister came over just like my in-law said she would. She took one look at me and started praying. Not the kind of gentle, whisper prayers you hear in church sometimes. This was the kind of prayer that commands mountains to move, the kind that reminds the devil he's already lost, the kind that calls things that are not as though they were.

She prayed over me, and I felt something break. Not break like breaking down—break like breaking free. Like chains I didn't even know I was wearing suddenly fell off and hit the floor.

"You're going to be alright," she said, holding my face in her hands. "Don't let this thing get to you, girl. You're going to be alright."

And for the first time since the diagnosis, I believed it might be true.

That was the day I made a decision. Not a decision to be perfect, not a decision to pretend MS wasn't real, not a decision to put on a brave face and act like everything was fine. I made a decision to fight. I made a decision to live. I made a decision to find out what Eunice Newton was made of when life tried to break her.

I didn't know then that this decision would lead me to write this book. I didn't know it would lead me to become a voice for other people going through their own battles. I didn't know it would teach me things about

CHAPTER 1: THE DAY I GOT UP

faith and strength and community that I never would have learned otherwise.

All I knew was that I was tired of being tired. I was tired of letting fear make my decisions. I was tired of my kids seeing their mama as someone who had given up instead of someone who got up.

So I got up.

I got up and decided that MS might be in my body, but it wasn't going to be my story. I got up and decided that I was going to learn everything I could about this condition and figure out how to live with it instead of just surviving it. I got up and decided that if I was going through this, then maybe I could help somebody else who was going through it too.

I got up and decided to live.

Not just exist, not just make it through each day, but really live. Live with purpose, live with joy, live with the knowledge that sometimes the worst thing that happens to you can become the thing that reveals who you really are.

That Sunday morning changed everything because it was the morning I remembered something I had forgotten: I am not what happens to me. I am what I choose to do with what happens to me.

MS happened to me. But getting up? That was my choice.

And every morning since then, I make that same choice. Some days it's easier than others. Some days I wake up and my body reminds me real quick that I'm dealing with something serious. Some days the fatigue hits me like a truck and I have to use my cane or my scooter and people stare and I remember that my life looks different now than it used to.

But every day, I choose to get up.

Because that voice I heard that Sunday morning wasn't just talking about getting out of bed. It was talking about getting up in every sense of the word. Getting up and fighting. Getting up and living. Getting up and showing the world that you can't be counted out just because life tried to count you down.

If you're reading this book, chances are you're laying in your own bed right now—maybe literally, maybe figuratively—wondering if you can do it. Wondering if you're strong enough, brave enough, resilient enough to face whatever battle you're fighting.

Let me tell you what that voice told me: You can do it.

You can do it not because it's going to be easy, but because you're stronger than you know. You can do it not because you won't have bad days, but because bad days don't have to become a bad life. You can do it because getting up isn't about being perfect—it's about being persistent.

So whatever bed you're laying in right now—whether it's depression, illness, loss, fear, or just the overwhelming weight of life—I want you to hear what I heard that Sunday morning.

You can do it.

Now get up. We've got work to do.

"The moment you decide to get up is the moment your comeback begins. It's not about the bed you're in—it's about the choice you make to get out of it." - E.N.

CHAPTER 2

BEFORE THE BREAKDOWN

You know, people always want to know what life was like before. Before the diagnosis, before the hospital stay, before everything changed. They ask like maybe if they can understand what "normal" looked like, they can figure out how to protect their own normal from disappearing overnight.

I get it. I used to be the same way when I heard about other people's struggles. I'd listen to their stories and think, "But what were you doing before this happened? What could you have done differently?" Like there was some magic formula that could keep the storms of life from reaching my door.

But here's what I've learned: there is no before and after when it comes to who you are at your core. There's just different chapters of the same story. And my story has always been about movement, about not staying still, about showing up for the people I love even when—especially when—it's hard.

Before MS, I was Tweety from Harlem. I was the girl everybody knew, the one who was always on the go, always doing something, always available when someone needed help. I was a teaching assistant, which meant I was on my feet all day, walking from classroom to classroom, bending down to help kids with their work, running around making sure everybody had what they needed.

I loved that job. Loved those kids. There's something about working in education that feeds your soul, you know? Every day, you get to be part of someone's growth, someone's discovery, someone's breakthrough. I'd see a kid struggle with reading for weeks, then suddenly it would click, and their whole face would light up. That light—that was what got me up in the morning.

I had my routine down to a science. Wake up at 5 AM, get myself together, make sure my son had everything he needed for school, get to work by 7:30, stay until the kids were dismissed, then head home to start the evening routine—dinner, homework, baths, bedtime stories, a little time to myself if I was lucky.

On weekends, I was the mom at every basketball game, cheering loud enough for the whole gym to hear me. My son played basketball, and honey, I was his biggest fan. I'd travel to all his games, didn't matter how far. I'd pack snacks, bring my portable chair, and make sure that boy knew his mama was there supporting him no matter what.

I was also the friend who showed up. You know that friend—the one you call when you need someone to help you move, or when you're going through a breakup and need someone to sit with you and eat ice cream and talk trash about your ex, or when you just need someone to go to the lounge with you because you don't want to go alone. That was me. Always ready to show up, always ready to be there.

CHAPTER 2: BEFORE THE BREAKDOWN

My social calendar was packed. I'm talking packed. Lounges, parties, family gatherings, community events—if something was happening in Harlem, chances are I was going to be there. I loved being around people, loved the energy of a good party, loved getting dressed up and feeling beautiful and dancing until my feet hurt.

And honey, I could dance. Before MS, I had rhythm for days. I'd get on that dance floor and move like I didn't have a care in the world. Music was—still is—my thing. Put on some good music and I was transformed. It cleared my mind, lifted my spirit, made everything else fade away.

I was also the caretaker in my family. You know how it is—there's always that one person everyone calls when something needs to be handled. Need someone to take a family member to the doctor? Call Tweety. Need someone to help plan the family reunion? Call Tweety. Need someone to mediate an argument between relatives? Call Tweety.

I didn't mind it. Well, most of the time I didn't mind it. It felt good to be needed, to be the one people could count on. But looking back now, I can see that I was running myself ragged trying to be everything to everybody.

My days were long and full. I'd be at work all day on my feet, then come home and cook dinner, help with homework, clean the house, do laundry, make sure everybody had what they needed for the next day. Then I'd fall into bed exhausted, only to wake up the next morning and do it all over again.

But here's the thing—I loved it. I loved being busy, loved being needed, loved the feeling of accomplishment that came from taking care of my responsibilities and my people. I thought being tired at the end of the day meant I was living my life right.

I was healthy then, or at least I thought I was. Sure, I got tired sometimes, but who doesn't? Sure, my back hurt from being on my feet all day, but that seemed normal for someone who worked with kids. Sure, I sometimes felt a little off balance, but I chalked it up to wearing heels too much or just moving too fast.

The truth is, I wasn't paying attention to my body the way I should have been. I was so focused on taking care of everyone else that I wasn't really taking care of myself. I'd grab fast food instead of cooking healthy meals for myself. I'd stay up too late because that was the only time I had to myself. I'd push through pain or fatigue because there was always something that needed to be done.

I think a lot of us live like that, especially women, especially mothers. We're so busy being the glue that holds everything together that we don't notice when we're starting to come apart ourselves.

My relationship with food back then was... well, let's just say it wasn't great. I'd eat whatever was convenient, whatever was quick, whatever would give me energy to keep going. Fast food, processed food, whatever the kids wanted—I wasn't thinking about nutrition or how what I was eating might be affecting my body.

I drank sometimes too. Not like an alcoholic or anything, but I'd have drinks when I went out, maybe have some wine after a long day. It was social, it was fun, it was how I unwound. I had no idea that what I was putting in my body might be setting the stage for what was coming.

But you know what? I don't regret any of it. That busy, full, complicated life taught me things I needed to know. It taught me how to prioritize, how to multitask, how to show up for people even when I was tired. It taught me the value of community, the importance of being present for the people you love, the joy that comes from being needed and useful.

Most importantly, it taught me that I was stronger than I thought I was. All those years of juggling work and motherhood and relationships and community obligations—that was training. I just didn't know what I was training for yet.

See, I think sometimes God prepares us for battles we don't even know are coming. All those years of getting up early and staying up late, of pushing through when I was tired, of finding solutions to problems that seemed impossible—that was building my resilience muscle. I was learning how to handle hard things, how to keep going when keeping going felt impossible.

I was also building my support system, though I didn't realize it at the time. Every relationship I invested in, every time I showed up for someone else, every connection I made in my community—all of that was creating a network of people who would show up for me when I needed them most.

My kids were watching too. Every time I got up early to make sure they had what they needed, every time I showed up to their games and events, every time I kept going even when I was tired—I was showing them what it looked like to be resilient, to be dependable, to be someone who doesn't give up.

I didn't know I was teaching them these lessons. I thought I was just being a mom. But when MS hit and I had to learn how to fight for my life, they already knew what their mama was made of because they'd been watching me fight for them their whole lives.

The woman I was before MS wasn't perfect. She was tired sometimes, overwhelmed sometimes, probably too busy for her own good. She made mistakes, ate too much fast food, didn't go to the doctor as often as she should have, probably said yes to too many things and no to too few.

But she was also strong. She was loving. She was resilient. She was a fighter, even if she didn't know she'd need those fighting skills for herself one day.

And when everything changed, when MS entered the picture and turned my world upside down, all of those qualities I'd developed over the years didn't disappear. They went underground for a while during the darkest days, but they were still there, waiting for me to remember who I was.

That's what I want you to understand if you're going through your own battle right now. The person you were before this thing happened to you—that person is still in there. All the strength you've shown, all the love you've given, all the times you've gotten up and kept going—those weren't accidents. Those were you becoming who you needed to be for this moment.

Your "before" wasn't a separate life that's gone forever. Your "before" was preparation for your "now."

And the woman who could handle all of that—the busy days, the sleepless nights, the constant demands, the endless responsibilities—that woman is strong enough to handle whatever comes next.

Trust me on this one. I know her personally.

"Your past isn't something you lost when life changed—it's the foundation you're building your comeback on." - E.N.

CHAPTER 3

SIGNS I CHOSE TO IGNORE

Your body talks to you long before it has to scream.

I know that now. But back then, when the signs first started showing up, I was too busy, too distracted, too convinced that I was invincible to listen. I think that's how it happens for most of us. Life gets loud, responsibilities pile up, and we learn to push through discomfort because stopping isn't an option.

But your body? Your body keeps receipts. And eventually, it's going to demand that you pay attention.

The first sign I remember was the twitching. My right leg would twitch like it had a mind of its own. I'd be sitting at my desk at work, or laying in bed at night, and suddenly my leg would start jumping like someone was sending little electrical shocks through it.

I ignored it.

I told myself it was stress. I told myself it was because I'd been on my feet all day. I told myself it was nothing, because nothing was what I had time for it to be. I had kids to take care of, a job to do, a life to live. I didn't have time for mysterious leg twitches that probably didn't mean anything anyway.

Then came the balance issues.

I'd be walking down the hallway at work, same hallway I'd walked down hundreds of times, and suddenly I'd feel... off. Like the ground wasn't quite where I expected it to be. Like my body wasn't quite following the directions my brain was giving it.

The first time it happened, I looked around to see if anyone noticed. They didn't. So I kept walking, told myself I was just tired, maybe didn't eat enough breakfast, maybe my blood sugar was low. There was always an explanation that made more sense than something being wrong with me.

But it kept happening.

I'd be walking with my son, and suddenly I'd have to reach out and touch the wall to steady myself. Or I'd be walking to the store, and I'd feel like I might stumble for no reason at all. My son would look at me sometimes with this concerned expression, like he was seeing something I wasn't ready to see yet.

"You okay, Mom?"

"I'm fine, baby. Just moving too fast."

Always an excuse. Always a reason that had nothing to do with my body trying to tell me something important.

CHAPTER 3: SIGNS I CHOSE TO IGNORE

The balance problems got worse when I was pregnant with my son. I was about six months along when I really started noticing that something felt different. But I was pregnant—of course I felt off balance. I was carrying extra weight, my center of gravity was changing, my hormones were all over the place. That explained everything, right?

After he was born, the symptoms went away for a while. See? I told myself. It was just the pregnancy. Nothing to worry about.

But then he turned six months old, and everything came back harder than before.

The twitching wasn't just occasional anymore. The balance issues weren't just when I was tired. And now there was something new—a weakness in my right leg that made it feel like it wasn't fully mine anymore.

I'd be walking, and suddenly my right leg would feel heavy, like I was dragging it behind me instead of stepping with it. I'd be going up stairs, and my right leg would shake with the effort of lifting my body weight.

Still, I found ways to explain it away.

I was a new mom. I was sleep deprived. I was probably not eating right. I was probably pushing myself too hard trying to do everything. It was stress. It was fatigue. It was anything except what it actually was.

The truth is, I was scared to face what it might be. You know how it is when you suspect something might be really wrong, but acknowledging it makes it real? I was living in that space between knowing and not knowing, where you can still pretend everything is fine as long as you don't look too closely.

But my body wasn't letting me pretend anymore.

At work, my coworkers started noticing. These were people who saw me every day, who knew how I normally moved, how I normally carried myself. And they were seeing changes I was still trying to deny.

My boss was the one who finally said something. I remember that morning so clearly. It was a Monday or Tuesday, just a regular day, and I was walking to my desk like I did every morning. But I was limping. Not dramatically, not obviously, but enough that someone who cared about me would notice.

He came over to my desk and said, "That's not normal."

Those three words hit me like a punch to the stomach because I knew he was right. It wasn't normal. None of it was normal. But I'd been working so hard to make it seem normal, to myself and everyone else, that hearing someone else say it out loud felt like having a light shined on something I'd been keeping in the dark.

"You need to check yourself into the hospital on Friday," he said. "See what's going on, because I don't like the way you're limping all the time. You're too young for that."

I wanted to argue with him. I wanted to say I was fine, that it was nothing, that he was overreacting. But I couldn't, because deep down, I knew he wasn't.

Even then, even with my boss telling me to go to the hospital, I tried to minimize it. I went to one of those quick care places first, hoping they'd tell me it was something simple. Maybe I needed vitamins. Maybe I needed to rest more. Maybe I needed to change my shoes.

CHAPTER 3: SIGNS I CHOSE TO IGNORE

They told me it was probably low iron. See? Nothing serious. Just low iron. I could take some supplements and everything would go back to normal.

But it didn't.

If anything, the symptoms got worse. The weakness in my leg became more pronounced. The balance issues became more frequent. And now there was pain—not just discomfort, but real pain that would shoot through my right side like lightning.

I kept working. I kept taking care of my kids. I kept pushing through because that's what I'd always done. Push through the tiredness, push through the stress, push through whatever obstacle was in my way.

But this wasn't an obstacle I could push through.

The day I finally went to the hospital—the day that would change everything—I was in severe pain. The kind of pain that makes you nauseous, that makes you break out in a cold sweat, that makes you realize you can't pretend anymore that nothing is wrong.

It was late at night when I finally admitted to myself that I needed help. I'd been in pain all day, but I'd been hoping it would pass, hoping I could sleep it off, hoping that tomorrow I'd wake up and feel normal again.

But as I lay in bed that night, the pain getting worse instead of better, I knew I couldn't wait anymore. I knew that all those signs I'd been ignoring, all those symptoms I'd been explaining away, all those moments when my body was trying to tell me something—they were leading to this moment.

I was scared. Scared of what they might find, scared of what it might mean, scared of how my life might change if this was something serious.

But I was also tired. Tired of hurting, tired of pretending, tired of carrying this fear around like a secret I couldn't tell anyone.

So I went.

And in those moments in the emergency room, waiting for test results, I thought about all the signs I'd ignored. The twitching that started years ago. The balance issues during pregnancy that I blamed on being pregnant. The weakness that got worse after my son was born. The pain that kept getting stronger no matter how much I tried to push through it.

I thought about how many times my body had tried to get my attention, and how many times I'd turned away because I was too busy, too scared, or too convinced that acknowledging the problem would make it worse.

Here's what I want you to understand: ignoring the signs doesn't make them go away. It just means you lose precious time that could have been spent getting help, getting treatment, getting support.

I'm not saying this to make you paranoid about every ache and pain. I'm saying this because I learned the hard way that our bodies are smarter than we give them credit for. When something is wrong, really wrong, your body will keep sending you messages until you listen.

The twitching, the balance issues, the weakness, the pain—these weren't random things happening to me. They were my body's way of saying, "Pay attention. Something needs to be addressed. Don't ignore me."

CHAPTER 3: SIGNS I CHOSE TO IGNORE

I ignored those messages for months, maybe years. And while I can't say for certain that earlier intervention would have changed my diagnosis, I can say that all that time I spent afraid and in denial was time I could have spent getting answers, getting treatment, getting the support I needed.

If you're reading this and you're ignoring signs from your own body—strange symptoms you can't explain, pain that won't go away, changes that worry you but that you keep telling yourself are nothing—please don't do what I did.

Please listen.

Your body isn't your enemy. It's not trying to inconvenience you or ruin your plans. It's trying to take care of you the only way it knows how—by getting your attention when something needs attention.

Don't wait until the whispers become screams. Don't wait until you're in the emergency room at midnight, wishing you'd acted sooner.

Listen to your body. Trust your instincts. Get the help you need.

Because the signs you're ignoring today might be the lifeline you need tomorrow.

"Your body doesn't lie to you—it just waits patiently for you to stop lying to yourself." - E.N.

PART II: THE DIAGNOSIS

CHAPTER 4

FIVE DAYS THAT CHANGED MY LIFE

I went to the hospital thinking I'd get some medicine and go home.

That's how naive I was about what was happening to my body. Even with all the signs I'd been ignoring, even with the pain that had gotten so bad I couldn't sleep, even with my boss telling me something wasn't right—I still thought this was something that could be fixed with a prescription and a good night's rest.

It was around 10 o'clock at night when I finally admitted I couldn't wait any longer. The pain in my right side was so severe I was nauseous, sweating, struggling to even walk straight. I called my family, told them I was going to the emergency room, and tried to downplay how scared I was.

The ER at night is a different world. Harsh fluorescent lights, the smell of disinfectant mixed with fear, people in various states of crisis waiting for answers they're not sure they want to hear. I checked in, gave them my information, and settled in to wait.

But I didn't wait long.

The moment the triage nurse saw me trying to walk, she knew something was seriously wrong. I was limping badly, having to lean on things to stay upright, clearly in distress. They rushed me back immediately.

"We need to do some tests," the doctor said. "Based on what you're describing and what we're seeing, we want to get a better look at what's going on."

The first test was an MRI of my brain. Let me tell you, if you've never had an MRI, it's like being put into a very loud, very small tunnel while someone pounds on the outside with hammers. They give you headphones, but you can still hear everything—the thumping, the whirring, the mechanical sounds that seem to go on forever.

I lay there in that machine, trying to stay still, trying not to panic, trying not to think about why they needed to look at my brain. What were they looking for? What did they think was wrong with me?

When the test was over, they didn't tell me anything right away. Just said the doctor would review the results and be back to talk to me.

I waited. And waited. And waited.

You know how time moves differently in a hospital? How minutes feel like hours when you're waiting for news that might change your life? I kept checking the clock, kept looking toward the door, kept wondering what was taking so long.

CHAPTER 4: FIVE DAYS THAT CHANGED MY LIFE

Finally, the doctor came back. I'll never forget the look on his face—that careful, professional expression doctors wear when they have to deliver news they wish they didn't have to give.

"I'm sorry to let you know this," he said, "but you have MS."

MS. Two letters that meant nothing to me.

"What is that?" I asked. "What is MS?"

"Multiple Sclerosis," he said.

I stared at him. Multiple what? I'd never heard those words put together before. I had no idea what he was talking about, no frame of reference for what this meant for my life.

"Okay," I said, because I didn't know what else to say. "Like, what's the problem? Can this be cured? Can I just take some medicine and call it a day?"

That's when I saw it—that look doctors get when they have to explain that there's no quick fix, no magic pill, no going back to the way things were before.

"It's not curable," he said gently. "But it's treatable. We're going to admit you for five days so we can start you on steroids and begin a treatment plan."

Five days. In the hospital. For something I'd never heard of, something that couldn't be cured.

That's when it started to hit me that this wasn't a minor thing I could handle with some rest and medication. This was something bigger, something that was going to change my life in ways I couldn't even begin to understand yet.

They admitted me that night, and I called my family to let them know what was happening. I tried to sound calm, tried to act like everything was going to be fine, but I could hear the fear in my own voice.

"They're keeping me for five days," I told my mom. "Something called MS. Multiple Sclerosis. I don't really know what it means yet."

The first night in that hospital bed, I couldn't sleep. Not because of the pain—they'd given me something for that—but because my mind was racing. MS. Multiple Sclerosis. What did that mean for my kids? What did that mean for my job? What did that mean for my future?

I stared at the ceiling and tried to process what had just happened to my life.

The next morning, the doctors started explaining things to me. MS is an autoimmune disease where your immune system attacks the protective covering around your nerves. That's what was causing the weakness, the balance issues, the pain. My own body was attacking itself, and there was no way to make it stop completely.

They started me on high-dose steroids immediately. These weren't the kind of steroids athletes use—these were powerful anti-inflammatory medications designed to reduce the swelling around my nerves and hopefully improve my symptoms.

"The medication we're giving you is typically used for cancer patients," the doctor explained. "It's strong, but it's what we need to help manage your condition."

CHAPTER 4: FIVE DAYS THAT CHANGED MY LIFE

Cancer medication. For something I'd never heard of a week ago.

Each day in that hospital, I learned something new about MS. I learned that it's unpredictable—some people have mild symptoms, others become severely disabled. I learned that it often affects young adults, especially women. I learned that there's no cure, but there are treatments that can help slow its progression.

I learned that I would need to take medication for the rest of my life. Infusions twice a year of a powerful drug that would hopefully keep my immune system from doing more damage to my nerves.

But the hardest thing to learn was how much my life was going to change.

"You'll need to be careful not to overexert yourself," they told me. "Stress can trigger relapses. Heat can make symptoms worse. You'll need to pace yourself differently than you did before."

Pace myself differently. For someone who had never sat still, who prided herself on being able to handle anything, who defined herself by how much she could do—this felt like being told to become a different person.

Every day I was in that hospital, reality sank in a little deeper. This wasn't going away. This wasn't something I could push through or ignore or overcome through sheer willpower. This was my new normal, and I had to figure out how to live with it.

The doctors were kind, but they were also honest. They explained that MS affects everyone differently, so they couldn't predict exactly what my future would look like. Some people live relatively normal lives with minimal symptoms. Others end up in wheelchairs. Most people fall somewhere in between.

"The important thing," one doctor told me, "is that this doesn't mean your life is over. It means your life is different. But different doesn't mean worse—it just means you'll need to learn new ways of doing things."

By the third day, the reality was starting to settle in, and so was the depression. I wasn't just dealing with a medical diagnosis—I was dealing with the loss of the life I thought I was going to have. The loss of the person I thought I was. The loss of the future I had planned.

I spent a lot of time crying in that hospital bed. Crying for the woman who could work all day without getting tired. Crying for the mother who could keep up with her kids at the playground. Crying for the person who never had to think twice about her body's ability to do what she asked of it.

The nurses were wonderful. They'd come in and check on me, bring me tissues, sit with me when I needed someone to listen. But at the end of the day, I was alone with this diagnosis, alone with this new reality, alone with the fear of what came next.

By the fifth day, when they were getting ready to discharge me, I still felt like I was in a fog. They gave me a list of medications to take, a list of symptoms to watch for, a list of lifestyle changes to make. They scheduled follow-up appointments and gave me pamphlets about living with MS.

But I felt like I was being sent home to a life I didn't recognize, in a body I didn't understand, with a condition I still couldn't fully comprehend.

"You're going to be okay," the discharge nurse told me as she went over my instructions. "This is manageable. Lots of people live full, happy lives with MS."

CHAPTER 4: FIVE DAYS THAT CHANGED MY LIFE

I nodded and smiled because that's what you do when someone is trying to encourage you. But inside, I was terrified.

How was I supposed to tell my kids that Mommy had a disease that might get worse? How was I supposed to go back to work and pretend everything was normal? How was I supposed to live a full, happy life when I didn't even know what that looked like anymore?

Those five days in the hospital didn't just give me a diagnosis—they gave me a new identity I never asked for. I walked in as Tweety from Harlem who was having some health issues. I walked out as a woman with Multiple Sclerosis, with all the uncertainty and fear that came with those words.

But here's what I didn't know then, what I couldn't see in those early days when everything felt dark and scary and impossible: those five days weren't the end of my story. They were the beginning of a different chapter.

A chapter where I would learn what I was really made of. A chapter where I would discover strength I didn't know I had. A chapter where I would find out that having MS didn't mean I couldn't live—it just meant I had to learn how to live differently.

But all of that was still to come. In those first days after the diagnosis, all I knew was that everything had changed, and I had no idea how I was going to handle what came next.

"Sometimes the worst days of your life are actually the first days of who you're meant to become." - E.N.

CHAPTER 5

WHAT IS MS?

When someone tells you that you have a disease you've never heard of, your first instinct is to try to understand it. You want to know what it is, what it does, how it's going to affect your life. You want answers that make sense, explanations that help you feel like you have some control over what's happening to your body.

But sometimes the answers just make you more scared.

After I left the hospital, I did what most people do these days when they get a diagnosis they don't understand—I went looking for information. And let me tell you, that was both the best and worst thing I could have done.

The internet is full of information about MS, but not all of it is helpful, and some of it is downright terrifying. I read stories about people who went from walking to wheelchairs in a matter of years. I saw pictures of brain scans that looked like Swiss cheese. I read statistics about disability and progression and life expectancy that made my heart race and my palms sweaty.

But I also learned some things that helped me understand what was happening in my body, and why I'd been experiencing the symptoms that had brought me to the hospital in the first place.

Multiple Sclerosis—MS—is what they call an autoimmune disease. That means your immune system, which is supposed to protect you from infections and diseases, gets confused and starts attacking your own body instead. Specifically, it attacks something called myelin, which is like the protective coating around the wires in your nervous system.

Think of it like this: your nerves are like electrical wires, and myelin is like the plastic coating around those wires. When the coating gets damaged, the electrical signals don't travel properly. That's what causes the symptoms—the weakness, the balance problems, the twitching, the pain.

My doctor explained it to me like this: "Your body is basically short-circuiting in certain places. That's why you're having trouble with coordination and strength on your right side."

It made sense, in a terrifying way. All those months of symptoms I'd been ignoring—they weren't random. They were my nervous system trying to function with damaged wiring.

But here's what really got to me: nobody knows why it happens. They don't know what causes MS, they don't know why some people get it and others don't, and they don't know how to cure it. All they can do is try to slow it down and manage the symptoms.

"A lot of African Americans are getting it," my doctor told me when I asked where this came from. "We're actually doing research on MS now

CHAPTER 5: WHAT IS MS?

to figure out why, because we're seeing more cases in the Black community than we used to."

That didn't make me feel better. If anything, it made me feel like a statistic, like part of some medical mystery that nobody understood.

I asked everyone I could think of if they'd ever heard of MS. My family, my friends, people at work—most of them had never heard of it either. Or if they had, they knew someone who had it and the stories weren't always encouraging.

I had an uncle who had MS. I remembered seeing him suffer before he passed away, remembered how the disease had changed him, made him weaker, made it harder for him to do the things he used to love. That's what I had now. That's what I was facing.

But then I started hearing other stories too. My doctor told me about patients who were living full, active lives years after their diagnosis. I met people online who had MS and were still working, still traveling, still raising families. I learned that MS affects everyone differently, and that having it doesn't automatically mean your life is over.

"Everybody's body is different," my doctor kept telling me. "You might hear stories about your situation, but let me tell you something—you don't listen to those stories. Your body is different from others. You might hear stories that somebody might pass away, but you've got to ignore all that because your body is different."

That became my lifeline in those early days when I was trying to understand what having MS meant for my future. Your body is different.

Your experience is different. Don't let other people's stories determine your story.

But it was hard not to get scared when I learned about relapses—periods when symptoms get worse or new symptoms appear. It was hard not to worry when I read about people who went from walking to needing mobility aids. It was hard not to panic when I realized that this disease was unpredictable, that I might wake up one day and not be able to do things I could do the day before.

The medication they put me on was another reality check. Twice a year, I would need to go for infusions of a powerful drug that would hopefully slow down the progression of the disease. The same medication they give to cancer patients. That's how serious this was.

"It's a hard medication," the doctor explained. "But it's what we need to help manage your condition and hopefully prevent relapses."

I learned about the importance of avoiding stress, because stress can trigger relapses. I learned about avoiding heat, because heat can make symptoms worse. I learned about the need to pace myself, to listen to my body, to not push through fatigue the way I always had before.

All of this information was overwhelming, but it was also empowering in a way. For months, I'd been dealing with symptoms I couldn't understand. Now I had answers. Now I knew why my leg had been twitching, why I'd been losing my balance, why I'd been getting weaker.

It wasn't in my head. It wasn't because I was getting older or because I was stressed or because I wasn't taking care of myself well enough. It was a real, medical condition with a name and an explanation and a treatment plan.

CHAPTER 5: WHAT IS MS?

But knowing what it was didn't make it easier to accept.

I struggled with the word "chronic." MS is a chronic condition, which means it's not going away. Ever. This wasn't like having the flu or even breaking a bone—something that would heal and then be done. This was something I would have to manage for the rest of my life.

I struggled with the word "degenerative." While not everyone with MS gets worse over time, the disease can be progressive, meaning symptoms can worsen or new symptoms can develop. There was no guarantee that I would stay as functional as I was right after diagnosis.

I struggled with the uncertainty. Nobody could tell me exactly what my future would look like. Would I be able to keep working? Would I be able to keep up with my kids? Would I be able to live independently? All they could say was "we'll have to wait and see."

That uncertainty was almost harder to deal with than the symptoms themselves. I'm the kind of person who likes to have a plan, who likes to know what's coming so I can prepare for it. But with MS, there is no definitive plan. There's just treatment and hope and taking it one day at a time.

One thing that helped me was learning that MS is actually more common than I thought. About a million people in the United States have it. That meant I wasn't alone, even though it felt like it sometimes. There were other people out there figuring out how to live with this same diagnosis, facing the same fears, asking the same questions.

I also learned that research is ongoing, that new treatments are being developed all the time, that the outlook for people with MS is better now than it was even ten years ago. That gave me hope, even when everything else felt scary and uncertain.

But the most important thing I learned about MS in those early days was this: having it doesn't define who you are. It's something you have, not something you are.

It took me a while to understand that distinction, and even longer to believe it. But my doctor kept reinforcing it every time I saw her.

"You have MS," she would say. "But you are still you. You're still a mother, still a woman, still someone with dreams and goals and things you want to do with your life. MS is just something you have to factor in now."

Learning about MS was scary, overwhelming, and sometimes depressing. But it was also the beginning of understanding how to live with it. Because once you know what you're dealing with, you can start figuring out how to deal with it.

And that's exactly what I had to learn to do.

"Knowledge about your condition is power, but don't let that knowledge become a prison. Learn what you need to know, then focus on how you're going to live." - E.N.

CHAPTER 6

THE BREAKDOWN

I thought my life was over.

I don't say that lightly, and I don't say it for dramatic effect. I mean it literally. In the months after my diagnosis, I genuinely believed that the life I had known, the woman I had been, the future I had planned—all of it was gone, and what was left wasn't worth living.

The depression hit me like a freight train I never saw coming.

I'd dealt with sadness before, stress before, hard times before. But this was different. This was a darkness so complete it felt like being buried alive. This was a hopelessness so profound it made getting out of bed feel impossible, let alone getting through an entire day.

It didn't happen all at once. For the first few weeks after leaving the hospital, I tried to act normal. I went back to work, tried to keep up with my routine, told people I was fine when they asked how I was doing. But inside, I was falling apart piece by piece.

Every morning when I woke up, there would be a split second—just a split second—when I forgot. When my brain hadn't fully come online yet and I was just Tweety from Harlem getting ready to start another day. But then reality would crash back in, and I would remember: I have MS. I have a chronic, incurable disease. My life is never going to be the same.

That realization hit me fresh every single morning like I was learning it for the first time.

The physical symptoms were hard enough to deal with. My right leg felt weak and unreliable. My balance was off, making me feel unsteady even when I was just standing still. The fatigue was unlike anything I'd ever experienced—not just tired, but exhausted in my bones, like my body was running on empty all the time.

But the emotional pain was worse than the physical pain. So much worse.

I felt like I was grieving, and in a way, I was. I was grieving the loss of the woman I used to be. The woman who could work all day without getting tired. The woman who could dance all night. The woman who never had to think twice about whether her body would cooperate with what her mind wanted to do.

I was grieving the loss of my future. All the plans I'd made, all the things I'd assumed I'd be able to do as I got older—suddenly all of that was uncertain. Would I be able to keep working? Would I be able to travel? Would I be able to take care of my kids the way they needed me to?

I was grieving the loss of my identity. So much of who I was had been tied up in being the strong one, the reliable one, the one who could handle anything. Now I felt weak, unreliable, like I couldn't even handle my own life, let alone help anyone else with theirs.

CHAPTER 6: THE BREAKDOWN

The worst part was feeling like I was all alone with this. Even though I had family and friends who loved me, even though people were trying to be supportive, I felt like nobody could possibly understand what I was going through. How could they? They still had their health, their certainty, their normal lives. They could offer sympathy, but they couldn't offer understanding.

I started isolating myself. I stopped going out with friends, stopped attending family gatherings, stopped doing the social things that used to bring me joy. When people invited me places, I would make excuses. I was tired, I wasn't feeling well, I had other plans. The truth was, I couldn't bear the thought of pretending to be okay when I felt so broken inside.

I spent more and more time in bed. Not because I was physically unable to get up, though some days that was part of it, but because bed felt like the only safe place in the world. Under those covers, I could pretend the outside world didn't exist. I could hide from the reality of my diagnosis, from the fear of what was coming next, from the overwhelming task of figuring out how to live with this new normal.

My kids started noticing. How could they not? Their mama, who had always been the one moving around, taking care of things, making sure everyone was okay—suddenly I was the one who needed taking care of.

My eight-year-old son would come into my room and see me just laying there, day after day. "You okay, Mom?" he would ask, and I would lie and tell him I was just tired, that I would feel better soon. But I could see the worry in his eyes, the confusion about why his strong mama wasn't acting like herself anymore.

My daughter, who was in college, would call and I could hear the concern in her voice when I didn't sound like myself. She was dealing with her own stress and challenges, and here I was adding to her burden by falling apart.

The guilt was eating me alive. Not only was I dealing with this diagnosis, but I was failing the people who needed me most. I was supposed to be the rock, the foundation, the one who held everything together. Instead, I was crumbling, and my family was watching it happen.

I called my family members crying so many times during those months. My aunt, my mother-in-law, my brothers—I would call them in the middle of the day, sobbing, telling them I couldn't do it anymore. That I didn't want to be here anymore. That I just wanted to give up.

"I can't do this," I would tell them through my tears. "This is too hard. I don't know how I'm supposed to live like this."

They would try to encourage me, try to remind me of how strong I was, try to give me reasons to keep fighting. But their words felt like they were coming from very far away, like I was hearing them through thick glass.

The scariest part was when the thoughts of ending it all started coming. I'm not proud to admit this, but there were days when I genuinely considered suicide. Not because I wanted to die, exactly, but because I couldn't see how I was going to live. The future looked so bleak, so full of uncertainty and decline and limitation, that not having a future seemed like the better option.

I would think about my kids and feel guilty for even having those thoughts. But then I would think about what kind of mother I was going

CHAPTER 6: THE BREAKDOWN

to be able to be with this disease, what kind of burden I might become, and the guilt would spiral in the other direction.

It was a dark, dark time. Darker than I had ever experienced before, darker than I hope to experience again.

I stopped taking care of myself. I barely ate, and when I did eat, it was whatever was easiest—fast food, processed junk, anything that required minimal effort. I stopped exercising, stopped doing my hair, stopped wearing anything but pajamas or sweatpants. What was the point? Who was I trying to look good for? What did it matter if I was just going to get sicker anyway?

I stopped talking to God too, which was maybe the most telling sign of how far I had fallen. I had always been a spiritual person, had always found comfort in prayer and faith. But during those dark months, I felt like God had abandoned me. How could a loving God let this happen to me? How could He take away my health, my future, my sense of who I was, and expect me to just accept it?

I was angry at God, angry at my body, angry at life, angry at everyone who still had their health and their certainty and their normal problems. I was drowning in bitterness and self-pity and despair.

My family was scared. I could see it in their faces when they looked at me, hear it in their voices when they talked to me. This wasn't just about adjusting to a medical diagnosis anymore. This was about whether I was going to survive this emotionally and mentally.

There were days when I honestly didn't know if I would.

The woman who had always been known for her strength, her resilience, her ability to keep going no matter what—that woman was nowhere to be found. In her place was someone I didn't recognize, someone who felt weak and defeated and hopeless.

I had lost myself completely.

But here's the thing about rock bottom: it's solid. When you can't fall any further, when you've lost everything you thought you were and everything you thought you had, there's something to build on. There's something to push against.

I didn't know it then, during those dark months when I could barely get out of bed, but I was about to discover something important about myself. I was about to learn that the woman I thought I had lost was still there, buried under all that pain and fear and depression, waiting for the right moment to fight back.

I was about to learn that sometimes you have to completely fall apart before you can put yourself back together in a way that's even stronger than before.

But first, I had to hit bottom. And that's exactly where I was.

"Sometimes the breakdown isn't the end of your story—it's the clearing away of everything that was hiding your true strength." - E.N.

PART III: FIGHTING BACK

CHAPTER 7

CLAIMING MY FIGHT, NOT MY ILLNESS

The turning point didn't come all at once. It came in small moments, tiny shifts in thinking that eventually added up to a completely different way of seeing my situation. But if I had to pinpoint when things started to change, it was the day I decided I was tired of being tired.

I was laying in bed—again—staring at the ceiling, feeling sorry for myself, when I heard my own voice in my head say something that surprised me: "This is not who you are."

It wasn't a booming revelation or a moment of sudden clarity. It was more like a quiet recognition, like running into an old friend you hadn't seen in a while. The real me—the fighter, the woman who didn't stay down, the person who had survived everything life had thrown at her so far—she was still there. She had just been buried under all that fear and depression and self-pity.

But she was still there.

I sat up in bed and looked around my room. Really looked. I saw the mess I'd been living in—clothes everywhere, dishes on the nightstand, medicine bottles scattered around, the general chaos that comes from someone who has stopped caring about their environment because they've stopped caring about themselves.

"This is not who you are," I said out loud this time.

I got up and started cleaning. Not because I felt amazing or because all my problems were suddenly solved, but because I needed to do something—anything—that felt like taking control instead of letting everything control me.

As I cleaned, I thought about what my doctor had told me during one of my follow-up appointments: "You have MS, but MS doesn't have you."

At the time, I thought it was just something doctors say to make patients feel better. But standing there, picking up clothes and organizing medicine bottles, I started to understand what she meant.

MS was something that was happening in my body. But it wasn't my identity. It wasn't my whole story. It wasn't the most important thing about me, even though it felt like it had become the only thing about me.

I was still Eunice Newton. I was still Tweety from Harlem. I was still a mother, a friend, a woman with dreams and goals and things I wanted to do with my life. MS was just something I had to factor in now, not something that erased everything else about who I was.

That night, I made a decision that changed everything: I decided I wasn't going to claim this illness as my identity.

CHAPTER 7: CLAIMING MY FIGHT, NOT MY ILLNESS

Let me explain what I mean by that, because it's important.

I'm not talking about denial. I wasn't pretending I didn't have MS or that it wasn't affecting my life. The symptoms were real, the limitations were real, the need for treatment was real. I couldn't just wish it away or think positive thoughts and make it disappear.

But there's a difference between acknowledging something and claiming it. There's a difference between saying "I have MS" and saying "I am an MS patient." There's a difference between managing a condition and letting that condition manage you.

I decided I was going to have MS, but I wasn't going to be MS.

This shift in thinking didn't happen overnight, and it didn't make all my problems go away. I still had bad days, still dealt with symptoms, still worried about the future. But I started approaching everything differently.

Instead of waking up every morning and immediately thinking about how MS was going to limit my day, I started thinking about what I wanted to accomplish and then figuring out how to work around any limitations.

Instead of avoiding social situations because I was embarrassed about my condition, I started being honest with people about what I was dealing with while also making it clear that I was still the same person they had always known.

Instead of letting fear of the future paralyze me, I started focusing on what I could control today.

I started saying things like "It's a minor thing" when people asked about my MS. Not because it was actually minor—it was a major life change that affected everything. But because calling it minor in my own mind helped me keep it in perspective. It helped me remember that this was one part of my life, not the whole thing.

I started telling people "Don't claim it" when they talked about their own health struggles or challenges. Because I learned that the language we use about our problems affects how we experience those problems. When you claim something as your identity, you give it power over your entire life. When you acknowledge it as something you're dealing with, you maintain power over how you deal with it.

My spiritual life started coming back during this time too. I began to see my diagnosis not as God punishing me or abandoning me, but as a test of my faith and my strength. Maybe this was happening for a reason I couldn't understand yet. Maybe I was going through this so I could help other people who would go through it later.

I started praying again, but differently than before. Instead of asking God to take this away from me, I started asking Him to give me the strength to handle it. Instead of asking why this happened to me, I started asking what I was supposed to learn from it.

"God, if you gave me this, then you must think I'm strong enough to handle it," I would pray. "Help me prove you right."

I also started being more intentional about my support system. During my darkest days, I had isolated myself from the people who cared about me. Now I started reaching out again, but I was more honest about what I needed from them.

I told my family that I didn't want them to treat me like I was fragile or sick, but I also needed them to understand that some days were harder than others. I told my friends that I might not be able to do everything I used to do, but I still wanted to be included, still wanted to be part of their lives.

Most importantly, I started being honest with my kids about what was happening, but in a way that didn't scare them.

"Mommy has something called MS," I told my son. "It makes me tired sometimes and it makes it harder for me to walk sometimes. But it doesn't change how much I love you, and it doesn't mean I can't take care of you."

I wanted him to understand what was happening without making him worry that he was going to lose his mama. I wanted him to see that people could have challenges and still live full, happy lives.

The other thing that helped me reclaim my sense of self was getting back into activities that made me feel like me. Music had always been important to me, so I started listening to music again—really listening, not just having it on in the background. I would put on my headphones and let the music fill up all the space in my head that had been occupied by worry and fear.

I started cooking again too. Not just heating up whatever was convenient, but actually cooking—making meals that nourished my body and my soul. There was something therapeutic about chopping vegetables, seasoning meat, creating something good from basic ingredients.

I even started thinking about getting back to some of my social activities. Not everything I used to do—some things weren't realistic anymore—but I didn't have to become a hermit just because I had MS.

The biggest change, though, was in how I talked about my future. Instead of assuming the worst-case scenario, I started planning for the best-case scenario while preparing for challenges along the way.

Yes, MS was unpredictable. Yes, I might have relapses. Yes, some things might get harder over time. But I might also have years of stable health. I might respond well to treatment. I might be one of the people who lives a relatively normal life with minimal symptoms.

I couldn't know which scenario would be mine, so I decided to hope for the best while being prepared for whatever came.

This shift from claiming my illness to claiming my fight changed everything. It gave me back my sense of agency, my feeling that I had some control over my life and my future. It helped me remember that I was still the same person who had overcome challenges before, who had raised children and built relationships and made a difference in her community.

MS was just the latest challenge. It was a bigger challenge than most, and it was going to require different strategies than the ones I'd used before. But it was still just a challenge, not a death sentence for the woman I had always been.

I was still here. I was still fighting. I was still me.

And that was something worth claiming.

"The moment you stop claiming your illness and start claiming your fight is the moment you take your power back." - E.N.

CHAPTER 8

FAITH AND FAMILY GOT ME UP

I want to tell you about my cousin. Her name was important to my story, even though she's not here to tell hers.

She had lupus. Like me, she was dealing with an autoimmune disease that was unpredictable, that changed her life in ways she never expected, that made her feel like her body was betraying her. Unlike me, she kept her struggle mostly to herself. She felt ashamed, insecure about her condition, worried about how people would see her if they knew what she was dealing with.

She passed away at 38 years old, just eleven days before her 39th birthday. On January 16th—a date I'll never forget because it marked the day I realized how precious and fragile life really is, and how important it is to live it fully while you can.

Before she died, she sent me a text message that I still have saved on my phone. In that message, she told me she looked up to me. She said she was proud of how I wasn't letting my MS stop me from living my life. She said she wished she could be more like me, that she wished she had my strength to face her illness head-on instead of hiding from it.

That message broke my heart and filled it at the same time.

It broke my heart because here was this beautiful, strong woman who was suffering in silence, who felt like she couldn't be open about her struggle, who was fighting a battle all alone. It broke my heart that she passed away before she could find the courage to tell her story, before she could inspire other people the way she was inspiring me.

But it also filled my heart because it reminded me that even in my darkest moments, even when I felt like I was failing at everything, I was still showing strength that other people could see. Even when I couldn't see it myself, my cousin could see that I was fighting, that I wasn't giving up, that I was trying to live my life despite this diagnosis.

Her message became one of my biggest motivations for getting back up and staying up. If she looked up to me, then I had a responsibility to be worth looking up to. If my fight was giving her hope, then I needed to keep fighting—not just for me, but for her, and for everyone else who might be watching, who might need to see that it's possible to live with chronic illness without letting it destroy your spirit.

After she passed, I made a promise to myself and to her memory: I was going to tell my story. I was going to be open about my struggle. I was going to show people that you can have MS or lupus or any other chronic condition and still live a full, beautiful, powerful life.

CHAPTER 8: FAITH AND FAMILY GOT ME UP

I was going to do what she couldn't do—speak up, speak out, and let people know that having an invisible illness doesn't make you less valuable, less beautiful, or less worthy of love and respect.

But I couldn't have made that promise, couldn't have kept that promise, without my faith and my family holding me up.

My father was a deacon before he passed away. My uncle is a pastor. I come from a family where faith isn't just something you talk about on Sundays—it's something that gets you through Monday, Tuesday, and every other day of the week. It's something that holds you up when you can't hold yourself up.

During my darkest days, when I was laying in that bed thinking about giving up, it was my family's faith that kept me anchored. Even when I was mad at God, even when I couldn't pray for myself, I had people praying for me, believing for me, holding onto hope when I couldn't hold onto it myself.

My mother-in-law and her sister were the first one to sense that something was seriously wrong with me emotionally. That Sunday morning when I heard the voice telling me to get up, she called me right after, like she had some kind of spiritual radar that told her I needed to hear from family.

"I'm not used to you being in bed like this," she said. "You've been in that bed for days. Something's wrong."

She was right. Something was wrong, and it wasn't just the MS. I was losing myself, losing my will to fight, losing my connection to the person I had always been.

She sent her sister over to check on me, and when she walked into that room and saw me, she didn't just offer sympathy. She offered spiritual warfare.

My aunt-in-law prayed over me with the kind of authority that only comes from someone who has been walking with God for decades, someone who has seen Him move mountains and isn't about to let the devil steal her niece's joy without a fight.

She laid hands on me and rebuked the spirit of despair, the spirit of hopelessness, the lies that were telling me my life was over. She spoke life over me, spoke strength over me, spoke healing over me—not just physical healing, but emotional and spiritual healing too.

"You're going to be alright," she said, holding my face in her hands. "Don't let this thing get to you, girl. You're going to be alright."

And for the first time in months, I believed it might be true.

That's what family does when you're in crisis. They don't just offer thoughts and prayers—they show up. They speak truth into your situation. They remind you who you are when you've forgotten. They hold onto your faith when yours is shaky.

My brothers were my strength in different ways. When I would call them crying, ready to give up, they wouldn't just comfort me—they would challenge me.

"You don't let that get to you," my brother would say. "You can do it. You can fight this. You've got kids to worry about, you know?"

CHAPTER 8: FAITH AND FAMILY GOT ME UP

He was reminding me of my purpose, my reason for fighting. It wasn't just about me anymore. It was about showing my kids what resilience looks like, what it means to face adversity and come out stronger on the other side.

My kids were watching everything. They were seeing how their mama handled this challenge, and that was going to shape how they handled challenges in their own lives. Did I want them to learn that when life gets hard, you give up? Or did I want them to learn that when life gets hard, you get harder?

The choice was obvious, but making that choice daily, living that choice daily, was the hard part.

My spiritual support system extended beyond my immediate family too. I had friends who would pray with me, encourage me, remind me of God's promises when I couldn't remember them myself.

One friend connected me with a prayer group specifically for people dealing with health challenges. Being around other people who understood the spiritual battle that comes with physical illness was incredibly healing. We would pray for each other, share scriptures that gave us strength, and remind each other that our conditions didn't define us—our faith did.

I learned during this time that faith isn't about never having doubts or never being scared. Faith is about holding onto God even when you can't understand what He's doing, even when His plan doesn't make sense to you, even when you're angry at Him for allowing difficult things to happen.

I was definitely angry at God for a while. I couldn't understand why He would give me this diagnosis, why He would allow my life to be turned upside down, why He would let me suffer when I had been trying to live right and serve Him.

But eventually, I came to see my MS differently. Maybe God wasn't giving me this condition as a punishment. Maybe He was trusting me with it because He knew I was strong enough to handle it and use it for His glory.

Maybe my struggle was going to help someone else with their struggle. Maybe my story was going to be the encouragement someone else needed to keep fighting. Maybe God was preparing me to be a voice of hope for people who felt hopeless.

That shift in perspective changed everything. Instead of asking God "Why me?" I started asking "What now? How do you want to use this? What do you want me to learn from this?"

My faith gave me a sense of purpose in my pain. It helped me see that even the worst things that happen to us can be used for good if we let God work through them.

My family gave me practical support too. They didn't just pray for me—they showed up for me. When I couldn't get to appointments, someone would drive me. When I was too tired to cook, someone would bring food. When I needed to talk, someone would listen.

They treated me like I was still me, not like I was fragile or broken or different. They expected me to keep fighting, keep trying, keep being the strong woman they had always known me to be. Their expectations helped me live up to them.

CHAPTER 8: FAITH AND FAMILY GOT ME UP

But they also gave me grace when I couldn't be strong every day. They understood that this was a process, that healing—physical and emotional—doesn't happen overnight, that some days would be better than others.

The combination of faith and family created a safety net that caught me when I was falling and a launching pad that helped me get back up. I couldn't have done this alone. Nobody should have to face chronic illness alone.

If you're reading this and you're dealing with your own health challenge, your own crisis, your own dark night of the soul—please don't try to handle it by yourself. Reach out to your faith community, lean on your family, let people help you carry the load.

And if you don't have that kind of support system naturally, create one. Find a support group, connect with others who understand what you're going through, build relationships with people who will speak life into your situation when you can't speak it yourself.

You need people who will pray for you when you can't pray for yourself. You need people who will believe in your recovery when you can't believe in it yourself. You need people who will remind you who you are when illness tries to make you forget.

Faith and family got me up. They can get you up too.

"When you can't hold onto hope yourself, surround yourself with people who will hold onto it for you until you're strong enough to take it back." - E.N.

CHAPTER 9

THAT SUNDAY MORNING VOICE

You know that voice I told you about? The one that got me out of bed that Sunday morning and changed the trajectory of my entire life?

I want you to understand something important about that voice: it wasn't unique to me. It's not something only special people get to hear. It's not reserved for the strongest or the most faithful or the most deserving.

That voice is available to you too. Right now. Wherever you are, whatever you're facing, however long you've been stuck in your own version of that bed I was lying in.

The question isn't whether the voice is there. The question is: are you ready to listen?

Let me tell you what I've learned about that voice in the five years since I first heard it clearly enough to act on it.

The voice speaks in different languages.

For me that Sunday morning, it sounded like my father—the deacon who never let anything keep him down, who taught me through his example that faith and strength go hand in hand. It sounded authoritative and loving at the same time, firm but encouraging.

But I've heard it in other forms since then. Sometimes it sounds like my mother-in-law's intuition, calling me at exactly the moment I need to hear from someone who loves me. Sometimes it sounds like my aunt-in-law's prayers, breaking chains I didn't even know were holding me captive. Sometimes it sounds like my cousin who passed away, reminding me to live fully because she couldn't.

Sometimes it sounds like my kids needing me to be strong. Sometimes it sounds like my doctor reminding me that I have MS but MS doesn't have me. Sometimes it sounds like a friend refusing to let me isolate myself.

And most of the time—if I'm being really honest—it sounds like me. The real me. The part of me that has always been a fighter, that has always found a way through whatever life threw at her, that was not about to let MS be the thing that finally took her down.

The voice you need to hear might sound like any of these things. It might sound like a loved one who has passed away and would want you to keep going. It might sound like God speaking directly into your situation. It might sound like your own inner wisdom that knows you're stronger than whatever you're facing.

Listen for it. Trust it. It knows what you need to hear.

The voice tells you what you already know but have forgotten.

CHAPTER 9: THAT SUNDAY MORNING VOICE

When I heard "You can do it," that wasn't new information. I had been doing hard things my whole life. I had overcome obstacles before. I had been knocked down and gotten back up more times than I could count.

But in that moment of deep depression, I had forgotten all of that. I had forgotten who I was. I had forgotten what I was capable of. I had forgotten that I had a choice in how I responded to what was happening to me.

The voice didn't give me strength I didn't have. It reminded me of the strength I'd always had but had temporarily lost sight of.

That's what the voice does. It cuts through all the noise—the fear, the pain, the self-doubt, the despair—and reminds you of the truth about who you really are.

You are stronger than you think you are. You have survived everything life has thrown at you so far. You have overcome challenges before. You have resources you haven't tapped into yet. You have people who care about you. You have reasons to keep fighting.

These things are true whether you can feel them right now or not. The voice just helps you remember.

The voice requires action.

Here's the thing about that Sunday morning: hearing the voice wasn't what changed my life. Getting up was what changed my life.

I could have heard "You can do it" and rolled over and gone back to sleep. I could have heard it and thought "That's nice, but I'm too tired, too sick, too broken." I could have heard it and dismissed it as wishful thinking or desperation or my mind playing tricks on me.

But I didn't. I sat up. I looked around. I put my feet on the floor. I stood up.

Those were small actions, but they were actions. And action is what transforms a voice in your head into a change in your life.

The voice will come to you—I believe that with everything in me. But you have to be willing to do something with what it tells you. You have to be willing to take that first small step, even when you're not sure where it will lead.

You have to be willing to get up.

The voice isn't a one-time thing.

That Sunday morning wasn't the only time I needed to hear "You can do it." It was just the first time I really listened and acted on it.

Since then, I've needed that voice hundreds of times. Every time I have a bad day with symptoms and want to feel sorry for myself. Every time I'm worried about the future and tempted to catastrophize about worst-case scenarios. Every time I compare myself to who I used to be and feel sad about what I've lost.

The voice shows up in those moments too. Sometimes loud, sometimes quiet, but always there if I'm willing to listen for it.

"You can do it." "You're stronger than this." "This is just one day, not your whole life." "You've handled worse and made it through." "Your kids need you to keep fighting." "This story isn't over yet."

CHAPTER 9: THAT SUNDAY MORNING VOICE

The voice adapts to what I need to hear in that specific moment, but the core message is always the same: Keep going. You've got this. Don't give up.

The voice becomes your voice.

Here's the beautiful thing that happens when you listen to that voice enough times and act on what it tells you: eventually, it stops feeling like something outside of you speaking to you. It starts feeling like something inside of you speaking through you.

It becomes integrated into who you are. It becomes part of your internal dialogue, your automatic response to challenges, your default setting when things get hard.

Now, when something difficult happens, I don't have to wait for some external voice to tell me I can handle it. I already know I can because I've proven it to myself over and over again. The voice that used to come from outside—from my father, from God, from my loved ones—now comes from my own deep knowing of who I am and what I'm capable of.

That's the goal. Not to always need someone else to remind you of your strength, but to internalize that truth so deeply that it becomes unshakeable.

The voice is calling to you right now.

I don't know what you're facing as you read these words. I don't know what bed you're lying in—literal or metaphorical—or how long you've been there. I don't know what diagnosis you're dealing with, what loss you're grieving, what trauma you're processing, what fear is keeping you stuck.

But I know the voice is calling to you.

It's saying: "You can do it."

It's reminding you: "You're stronger than you think you are."

It's encouraging you: "Get up. Your life is waiting for you."

It might sound like someone you love. It might sound like God. It might sound like the part of you that refuses to be defeated.

But it's there. It's real. And it's telling you the truth about what's possible for your life if you're willing to listen and act.

So here's my question for you: What is the voice telling you to do right now?

What small action is it asking you to take? What first step is it encouraging you to make? What choice is it inviting you to consider?

Listen for it. Really listen. Quiet all the other noise in your head—the fear, the doubt, the reasons why you can't—and listen for that voice that knows better.

And when you hear it, do what it says.

Get up.

Not because you feel ready. Not because you have all the answers. Not because the path forward is clear or easy or guaranteed to work out.

Get up because that voice knows something you might have forgotten: you have what it takes to handle whatever comes next. You've been

CHAPTER 9: THAT SUNDAY MORNING VOICE

building strength your whole life for exactly this moment. You're capable of more than you realize.

Get up because staying down isn't serving you anymore. Get up because your story isn't finished yet. Get up because the world needs what you have to offer.

Get up because somewhere deep inside you, underneath all the pain and fear and exhaustion, there's a part of you that has been waiting for permission to fight back.

This is that permission.

The voice is calling. It's time to answer.

You can do it.

Now get up.

"The voice that calls you to rise isn't something you have to search for—it's something you have to be still enough to hear. And once you hear it, brave enough to follow." - E.N.

PART IV: LEARNING TO LIVE AGAIN

CHAPTER 10

WHAT DOES MS LOOK LIKE?

"You don't look like you have MS."

I can't tell you how many times people have said that to me. They look at me with confusion, like they're trying to solve a puzzle that doesn't make sense. They see me walking around, taking care of my business, living my life, and they can't reconcile that with whatever they think MS is supposed to look like.

Every time someone says it, I ask them the same question: "What does MS look like?"

And you know what? They never have an answer.

That's because there is no look. There's no MS uniform, no special appearance that announces to the world that you're dealing with a chronic illness. MS doesn't care if you're beautiful or ugly, young or old, black or white, rich or poor. It doesn't change your face or make you wear a sign around your neck.

But people expect it to.

I think that's because most people only know about chronic illness from what they see in movies or on TV shows, where sick people look sick. They're pale and thin and obviously struggling. They're in hospital beds or wheelchairs, looking fragile and pitiful, inspiring everyone around them with their brave acceptance of their tragic fate.

That's not real life. That's definitely not my life.

Real life is more complicated than that. Real life is me getting dressed up to go out with my friends, walking with my cane, and having people tell me I'm "so pretty" like they're surprised that someone with MS could be attractive. Real life is me using my scooter to get around the city and having people stare at me like they're trying to figure out what's "wrong" with me.

Real life is having an invisible illness in a world that only recognizes visible ones.

Don't get me wrong—I'm grateful that my MS doesn't show on my face. I'm grateful that I can still get around, still take care of myself, still participate in life in meaningful ways. I know that not everyone with MS is as fortunate as I am, and I don't take that for granted.

But there's something isolating about dealing with a condition that people can't see. When you look "normal," people expect you to be normal. They expect you to have the same energy, the same capabilities, the same limitations as everyone else. And when you can't meet those expectations, they don't understand why.

I've had people get impatient with me for walking too slowly, not knowing that my right leg feels weak and unsteady, that every step requires more effort than it used to. I've had people question why I need to use a scooter for long distances, not understanding that what looks like a short walk to them feels like a marathon to me on bad days.

I've had people suggest that maybe I'm just lazy, or making excuses, or being dramatic about my symptoms. "You look fine," they say, like looking fine means feeling fine, like appearance equals reality.

But here's what I've learned about living with an invisible illness: just because people can't see your struggle doesn't mean it isn't real. Just because you don't fit their idea of what sick looks like doesn't mean you aren't dealing with something serious. Just because you're still functioning doesn't mean you aren't fighting a battle every single day.

MS affects everyone differently. Some people end up in wheelchairs, some people use walking aids, some people look completely normal but deal with crushing fatigue, cognitive issues, or pain that no one can see. Some people have good days and bad days. Some people have good years and bad years.

I fall somewhere in the middle of that spectrum. I use a cane when I'm walking short distances because it helps with my balance and gives me confidence. I use my scooter when I'm going longer distances because my leg gets weak and I don't want to risk falling or exhausting myself.

But most of the time, I just look like a regular woman going about her business. And that confuses people.

They see me at the grocery store, navigating the aisles with my scooter, and they look at me like I'm cheating somehow. Like I'm using a mobility aid I don't really need, taking advantage of accommodations meant for people who are "really" disabled.

They see me get up from my scooter to reach something on a high shelf, and I can practically hear them thinking, "I knew she was faking it." They don't understand that needing help with some things doesn't mean needing help with everything. They don't understand that disability isn't always all-or-nothing.

I've learned not to let other people's ignorance affect how I take care of myself. If I need my cane, I use my cane. If I need my scooter, I use my scooter. If I need to rest, I rest. If I need accommodations, I ask for them.

I don't owe anyone an explanation for how I manage my condition. I don't owe anyone proof that my illness is real or serious enough to warrant the help I need. I don't owe anyone a performance of suffering to make them comfortable with my reality.

What I do owe myself is the commitment to live my life as fully as possible, using whatever tools and resources I need to make that happen.

The truth is, most chronic illnesses are invisible. Depression, anxiety, lupus, fibromyalgia, Crohn's disease, diabetes, heart conditions, autoimmune disorders—millions of people are walking around looking "normal" while dealing with conditions that significantly impact their daily lives.

We've created a society that only recognizes and accommodates disability when it's obvious, when it fits our narrow definition of what suffering looks like. But that leaves out so many people who are struggling, who need support, who deserve understanding and compassion.

I want people to understand that you can be beautiful and sick at the same time. You can be strong and struggling at the same time. You can be grateful for what you have and still acknowledge what you've lost at the same time.

CHAPTER 10: WHAT DOES MS LOOK LIKE?

I want people to understand that when someone uses a mobility aid, they're not giving up or being lazy—they're being smart. They're conserving their energy for the things that matter most to them. They're choosing independence over pride, function over appearance.

I want people to understand that chronic illness doesn't follow the rules of acute illness. You don't get sick, get treatment, and get better. You learn to manage, to adapt, to find new ways of doing things. You have good days and bad days, sometimes good months and bad months. You celebrate small victories and grieve small losses.

But most of all, I want people to understand that having a chronic illness doesn't make you less valuable, less beautiful, less worthy of love and respect. It just makes you human in a way that's more visible, more obvious, than it is for people who haven't faced major health challenges yet.

Because here's the thing: we're all dealing with something. We're all fighting battles that other people can't see. We all have limitations, fears, struggles that we carry around invisibly.

The difference is that some of us have been forced to confront our mortality, our fragility, our humanity in a more direct way. Some of us have had to learn earlier than others that life is precious and unpredictable, that health is a gift not a guarantee, that strength comes in many different forms.

That's what MS looks like on me. It looks like someone who has been through something hard and came out stronger. It looks like someone who knows the value of every good day because she's experienced plenty of bad ones. It looks like someone who doesn't take her abilities for granted because she knows how quickly things can change.

It looks like resilience. It looks like adaptability. It looks like refusing to let circumstances define your worth or limit your joy.

It looks like me, getting up every day and choosing to live my life fully, using whatever tools I need to make that happen, not asking permission from anyone to take care of myself in the ways that work for me.

That's what MS looks like. It looks like life—messy, complicated, beautiful, challenging life—being lived by someone who refuses to be reduced to a diagnosis.

So the next time you see someone using a mobility aid who doesn't look sick enough to need it, the next time you encounter someone dealing with an invisible illness, the next time you're tempted to judge someone's reality based on their appearance—remember that you don't know their story.

Remember that strength comes in many forms, that disability looks many different ways, that some of the strongest people you'll ever meet are the ones who are fighting battles you can't see.

Remember that what chronic illness looks like, most of the time, is exactly like what health looks like—because we're all just people trying to live our lives the best way we know how.

"Don't assume you know someone's story based on how they look. The strongest battles are often the ones no one can see." - E.N.

CHAPTER 11

THIS BODY MAY BE SLOWER, BUT THIS SPIRIT IS FIRE

Let me tell you what my day looks like now, five years after my diagnosis, and how different it is from what it used to be.

I wake up at 5 AM, just like I always have. That part hasn't changed. I've always been a morning person, always liked to get up early and start my day before the world gets too loud and busy. But now, instead of jumping out of bed and hitting the ground running, I take a moment to check in with my body.

How do I feel today? Is my right leg stronger or weaker than yesterday? Am I dealing with fatigue that feels like I'm moving through thick honey, or do I have decent energy? Is my balance steady, or do I need to be extra careful today?

This isn't self-pity or dwelling on symptoms. This is practical planning. This is me being smart about how I'm going to navigate the next sixteen hours so I can accomplish what matters most to me without exhausting myself or putting myself at risk.

Some days, my body feels almost normal. I can walk without thinking about every step, move around my house without holding onto walls, feel like the woman I used to be. Those are good days, and I celebrate them.

Other days, my right leg feels heavy and uncooperative, like it belongs to someone else. My balance is off, and I have to move slowly and deliberately. The fatigue sits on my chest like a weight I can't lift. Those are harder days, but they're not bad days—they're just different days that require different strategies.

The biggest change in my daily routine is that I have to pace myself now. Before MS, I could work all day, take care of my family all evening, go out with friends all night, and bounce back the next day ready to do it all over again. My energy felt unlimited, like a well that never ran dry.

Now I have to budget my energy like I budget my money. I have to decide what's most important and make sure I save enough energy for those things. I can't do everything I used to do in a day, but I can still do the things that matter most to me.

For example, I still go to all of my son's basketball games. That boy is eight years old and playing his heart out, and I'm going to be there cheering for him no matter what. But now I use my scooter to get around the school, and I bring my portable chair so I don't have to stand for long periods. I plan the rest of my day around that game, making sure I don't wear myself out before the main event.

CHAPTER 11: THIS BODY MAY BE SLOWER, BUT THIS SPIRIT IS FIRE

I still cook for my family, because that's one of the ways I show love. But now I might sit on a stool while I'm chopping vegetables, or lean against the counter while I'm stirring pots. I've rearranged my kitchen so the things I use most often are within easy reach. I've learned to cook in batches when I'm feeling good, so I have meals ready when I'm not feeling as strong.

I still socialize with my friends, but differently than before. Instead of staying out until 2 AM dancing at the club, I might meet them for dinner or have them over to my house. I've had to educate my social circle about my limitations, but also about my capabilities. Yes, I need to sit down more often now. Yes, I might need to leave earlier than I used to. But I can still have fun, still enjoy good company, still be the person they've always known me to be.

The hardest adaptation has been around physical activity. I used to love to dance. Music would come on, and my body would just move, like it was having a conversation with the rhythm. Dancing was one of my favorite forms of self-expression, one of the ways I felt most like myself.

Now, my balance is too unpredictable for the kind of dancing I used to do. I tried it a few weeks ago when I went out with friends, and it just wasn't the same. My body couldn't keep up with what my spirit wanted to do, and that was hard to accept.

But you know what? Music still moves me. I still put on my headphones and let the music fill up all the empty spaces in my head. I still move to the rhythm, just differently now. Sometimes I dance sitting down. Sometimes I just close my eyes and let the music move through me without moving my body at all.

The spirit of dance—the joy, the freedom, the connection to something larger than myself—that's still there. It just looks different now.

That's become my philosophy about everything: the essence of who I am, the fire that drives me, the spirit that makes me who I am—none of that has changed. It just expresses itself differently now.

I'm still the woman who doesn't sit still, who has to stay busy, who needs to be productive to feel good about herself. But now staying busy looks like going to physical therapy twice a week instead of three times (they don't want me to overdo it and trigger a relapse). It looks like doing catering work from home instead of doing deliveries all over the city. It looks like being selective about which activities I commit to, instead of saying yes to everything.

I'm still the friend who shows up for people, but now I show up differently. Instead of being the one who helps you move apartments, I might be the one who brings food to your new place. Instead of being your dance partner at the club, I might be your conversation partner at dinner. I'm still there, still present, still offering support—just in ways that work with my current capabilities.

I'm still the mother who's involved in her children's lives, but I've had to be honest with them about my limitations and creative about working around them. When my son has basketball practice across town, his father takes him if I can't make it—we've been together over 23 years, and he's just as committed to our kids as I am. When my daughter needs help with something physical, I might ask her brother or her father to handle it.

CHAPTER 11: THIS BODY MAY BE SLOWER, BUT THIS SPIRIT IS FIRE

But I'm also teaching them things I couldn't teach them when I was healthy: how to be resilient in the face of challenges, how to adapt when circumstances change, how to ask for help when you need it, how to appreciate good days because you know how precious they are.

My kids are learning that strength isn't about being able to do everything yourself. It's about figuring out how to get things done even when you can't do them the way you used to. They're learning that love doesn't depend on physical capability, that being present emotionally is just as important as being present physically.

The thing that hasn't changed at all is my determination. If anything, that's gotten stronger. When you're forced to work harder for things that used to be easy, when you have to be more intentional about how you spend your energy, when you have to fight for every good day—you develop a level of determination that healthy people never have to access.

I am more determined now than I ever was before MS. Determined to live fully, to squeeze every drop of joy out of life, to make the most of whatever time and energy I have. Determined to show my kids what it looks like to thrive in spite of challenges. Determined to be an example for other people who are dealing with their own struggles.

My body may be slower now, but my spirit is on fire. My physical capabilities may be limited, but my emotional and spiritual capabilities feel limitless. My energy may be finite, but my love, my hope, my determination to make a difference in the world—those feel infinite.

People sometimes ask me if I miss the old me, the woman I was before MS. The honest answer is yes and no.

I miss the physical freedom I used to have. I miss being able to dance the way I used to dance, to walk as far as I used to walk, to have energy that felt unlimited. I miss the simplicity of not having to think about my body's limitations when making plans.

But I don't miss the woman who took her health for granted, who thought she was invincible, who didn't fully appreciate how precious every good day is. I don't miss the woman who was so busy being strong for everyone else that she forgot to take care of herself. I don't miss the woman who thought asking for help was a sign of weakness.

The woman I am now is more intentional, more grateful, more aware of what really matters. The woman I am now knows how to prioritize, how to say no to things that don't serve her, how to say yes to things that feed her soul. The woman I am now has been tested and proven, has been broken down and built back up stronger.

This body may be slower than it used to be, but this spirit—this spirit is fire. This spirit burns brighter because it's been through the refining process of struggle. This spirit knows its own strength because it's been forced to use every ounce of it.

This spirit refuses to be limited by physical circumstances. This spirit finds ways to dance even when the body can't keep up with the music. This spirit finds ways to shine even when the world tries to dim its light.

MS changed my body, but it couldn't touch my spirit. And as long as my spirit is still on fire, I'm still fully alive.

"When life slows down your body, let it speed up your appreciation for every moment you're still here to experience." - E.N.

CHAPTER 12

MY KIDS ARE MY PULSE

When I was in that dark place after my diagnosis, laying in bed day after day, my kids were the ones who kept checking on me. My eight-year-old son would come into my room with those big, worried eyes and ask, "Mommy, you okay?"

I would lie and tell him yes, but I could see that he knew something was wrong. Kids have this intuition about their parents, this ability to sense when the person who's supposed to be their rock is actually crumbling. And watching him worry about me, seeing the confusion on his little face when his always-moving mama was suddenly always in bed—that broke my heart in a way that even the MS diagnosis couldn't.

That's when I realized I had a choice to make. I could continue to let this illness destroy me, and in doing so, teach my children that when life gets hard, you give up. Or I could figure out how to fight this thing, and show them what it looks like to be resilient, to be strong, to keep going even when keeping going feels impossible.

The choice was obvious. My kids needed to see their mama be a fighter, not a victim.

I have three children—two daughters and one son. My oldest daughter is twenty years old and about to graduate from college next year. She's studying to be a doctor, which makes me incredibly proud and also a little nervous because I see how hard she's pushing herself, how much pressure she puts on herself to be perfect.

My middle daughter is in high school, dealing with all that teenage drama and figuring out who she wants to be in the world. She's at that age where she's watching everything I do, learning how to be a woman from watching how I handle being a woman.

And my son, my baby boy, is eight years old now. He was born right before my symptoms got really bad, so in a lot of ways, he's only known his mama as someone who deals with MS. But he's also seen his mama refuse to let MS defeat her.

Each of my kids has responded to my diagnosis differently, and each of them has taught me something important about resilience, about love, about what it means to be a family.

My oldest daughter was in college when I got diagnosed. She was dealing with her own stress and challenges, trying to figure out her future, managing the pressure of pre-med courses, and then she gets a call from home that her mama has a chronic illness that nobody really understands.

I felt so guilty about adding to her burden. Here she was, trying to build her own life, and now she had to worry about whether her mama was

CHAPTER 12: MY KIDS ARE MY PULSE

going to be okay. I tried to downplay it at first, tried to act like it wasn't a big deal, but she's too smart for that.

"Mama," she said during one of our phone calls, "you don't have to pretend with me. I know this is serious. But I also know you're strong enough to handle it."

That conversation meant everything to me because it reminded me that I had raised a daughter who could see my strength even when I couldn't see it myself. She had been watching me her whole life, learning how to be resilient by watching me be resilient, and now she was giving that strength back to me when I needed it most.

But she was also scared. I could hear it in her voice when she would call to check on me. She was worried about her grades slipping because she was distracted thinking about me. She was worried about what would happen if I got sicker. She was worried about having to take care of me instead of focusing on her own dreams.

That's when I had to have one of the hardest conversations of my life with her. I had to tell her that her job was to be my daughter, not my caretaker. Her job was to focus on her education, her future, her own life. My job was to take care of myself and manage my condition so that she could do exactly that.

"I didn't raise you to worry about me," I told her. "I raised you to be strong, to go after your dreams, to build the life you want. That's how you honor me—by living your life fully, not by putting your life on hold to take care of mine."

It took some time, but she finally understood what I meant. Now when she calls, she tells me about her classes, her goals, her plans for the future. She asks about my health, but she doesn't let worry about me dominate her life. She's learned to trust that I'm handling my business so she can handle hers.

My middle daughter, the one in high school, has been my toughest teacher. Teenagers don't have much patience for weakness, real or perceived. They need their parents to be strong, consistent, reliable. And here I was, dealing with a condition that made me unreliable sometimes, that meant I couldn't always be the parent she needed me to be in the exact way she needed me.

She was angry at first. Angry that I was sick, angry that our family life had to change, angry that she couldn't depend on me the way she used to. She would get frustrated when I had to use my cane or my scooter, embarrassed by the visible signs of my condition.

"Why can't you just be normal?" she asked me one day during a particularly difficult moment.

That question stung, but it also clarified something for me. I realized I had been so focused on managing my own feelings about having MS that I hadn't really helped my children process their feelings about it.

So I sat her down and we talked—really talked—about what was happening in our family.

"I know this is hard," I told her. "I know it's not what you wanted, and it's not what I wanted either. But this is our reality now, and we can either fight it together or let it tear us apart."

CHAPTER 12: MY KIDS ARE MY PULSE

I explained to her that I was still the same mama who loved her fiercely, who believed in her completely, who would do anything for her. I was just a mama who happened to have MS now, and that meant we had to do some things differently.

Slowly, she started to understand. She started to see that I was still strong, just strong in a different way. She started to see that asking for help when you need it isn't weakness—it's wisdom. She started to see that adapting to challenges is a life skill she was going to need whether I had MS or not.

Now she's one of my biggest supporters. She helps me when I need help, but she doesn't treat me like I'm fragile. She calls me out when I'm being stubborn about accepting assistance, but she also celebrates with me when I accomplish things that MS could have prevented me from doing.

But it's my son, my baby boy, who has been my greatest motivation through all of this.

He was so young when my symptoms really kicked in that he doesn't remember me being any different than I am now. To him, having a mama who uses a cane sometimes and a scooter sometimes is just normal. He doesn't see it as a limitation—he sees it as just another part of who I am.

He's also the one who keeps me moving. That boy plays basketball, and honey, I am not missing his games. I don't care if I have to roll up to that gymnasium in my scooter with my portable chair and my snacks—I'm going to be there cheering for him.

He sees me in the stands, and his whole face lights up. He waves at me between plays, points to me when he makes a good shot, looks for me in the crowd when he needs encouragement. He doesn't care that I'm the mama in the scooter—he just cares that I'm there.

And because he needs me to be there, I make sure I'm there. Because he's counting on me to show up, I show up. Because he believes his mama is the strongest woman in the world, I make sure I live up to that belief.

There was a day recently when my daughter was having a meltdown about school. She'd failed a test—got a 35 when she usually gets in the hundreds—and she was crying, telling me she couldn't do it, that she wanted to give up.

I looked at her and said, "You see your mama? You see me every day. I stop doing things for y'all? I stop being here, cooking, cleaning, going to basketball games, going to meetings? I'm always on the go, always doing things for y'all. So if I can do it, don't let that stop you. Take it over. Take that test over. You can do it. Don't let that stop you."

I reminded her that she's been watching me fight every single day. She's been watching me get up when I don't feel like getting up, push through when I want to give up, find ways to do things even when they're harder than they used to be.

"I'm a fighter," I told her, "and you're gonna fight too. You're gonna fight for that grade you want, for that career you want, for that life you want."

That's when I realized something important: my kids aren't just motivating me to keep fighting—they're learning how to fight by watching me fight. They're developing their own resilience by seeing mine in action.

My son sees me go to physical therapy twice a week, and he's learning that taking care of your body is important. My daughters see me advocate for myself with doctors, and they're learning that you have to speak up for what you need. All of them see me use mobility aids when I need them, and they're learning that using tools that help you is smart, not shameful.

They see me have bad days and good days, and they're learning that life isn't always easy, but you can still find joy in it. They see me adapt to challenges, and they're learning that flexibility is a strength, not a weakness.

Most importantly, they see me refuse to give up, and they're learning that giving up is never an option as long as you're still breathing.

My kids are my pulse because they keep my heart beating when everything else tries to make it stop. They're my motivation because I want them to be proud of how their mama handled this challenge. They're my teachers because they show me every day what unconditional love looks like.

They needed me to be strong, so I learned how to be strong. They needed me to keep going, so I learned how to keep going. They needed me to show them what resilience looks like, so I became resilient.

And now, watching them face their own challenges with the strength and determination they learned from watching me—there's no greater reward than that.

I didn't choose to have MS, but I did choose how to respond to it. And I chose to respond in a way that would make my children proud, that would teach them valuable lessons, that would show them that their mama is exactly as strong as they always believed her to be.

Because at the end of the day, that's what being a parent is about—not being perfect, but being present. Not avoiding all challenges, but showing your kids how to face them. Not having all the answers, but demonstrating how to keep looking for solutions.

My kids are my pulse, my heart, my reason for fighting. And as long as they need me to be strong, I'll find a way to be exactly that.

"Your children don't need you to be perfect—they need you to show them how to be resilient. They're watching how you handle life's challenges, and that becomes their blueprint for handling their own." - E.N.

PART V: FINDING PURPOSE IN PAIN

CHAPTER 13

FROM PAIN TO PURPOSE

The first time someone asked me about my MS, I was terrified.

I had been keeping my diagnosis mostly private for months, only telling close family and a few friends. I wasn't ready to be public about it, wasn't ready for the questions, the stares, the well-meaning but hurtful comments I knew would come.

But word gets around in a community like Harlem, especially when you're someone people know, someone who used to be everywhere and suddenly isn't around as much. People started noticing I was using a cane sometimes, that I moved differently than I used to, that something had changed.

The first person who asked me directly was someone I knew from the neighborhood. She saw me walking with my cane and said, "Hey, what's wrong? What happened to you?"

My heart started racing. This was the moment I'd been dreading—having to explain my situation to someone who wasn't family, having to say the words "I have MS" out loud to someone who might not understand, might judge me, might treat me differently afterward.

But I took a deep breath and told her the truth.

"I have MS," I said. "Multiple Sclerosis. It affects my nervous system, makes it harder for me to walk sometimes, makes me more tired than I used to be."

Instead of the pity or awkwardness I expected, she looked at me with genuine concern and said, "Oh wow, I'm sorry you're going through that. How are you handling it?"

And that's when something clicked for me. She wasn't looking at me like I was broken or tragic or someone to feel sorry for. She was looking at me like I was still me—just someone dealing with a challenge who might have something to teach her about handling challenges.

I found myself talking to her for twenty minutes about my experience, about what I'd learned, about how I was managing my symptoms and my emotions. And when we finished talking, she thanked me.

"You gave me hope," she said. "I've been dealing with some health issues too, and seeing how you're handling this makes me feel like I can handle mine."

That conversation changed everything for me. It was the first time I realized that my struggle could be someone else's strength, that my pain could have a purpose beyond just being something I had to endure.

CHAPTER 13: FROM PAIN TO PURPOSE

From that day forward, I started being more open about my MS. Not because I wanted attention or sympathy, but because I realized that hiding it wasn't helping anyone—not me, and not the people who might benefit from hearing my story.

The responses I got surprised me. Instead of treating me like I was fragile or different, most people respected my honesty and my strength. They asked thoughtful questions, shared their own struggles, thanked me for being real about what I was going through.

I started getting messages from people I hadn't heard from in years. Friends from high school, coworkers from old jobs, people from my community who had heard about my diagnosis and wanted to reach out.

Some of them had their own health challenges they'd been dealing with in silence. Some of them had family members with chronic illnesses. Some of them were just scared about their own mortality and found comfort in seeing someone they knew face a serious diagnosis with grace and determination.

One message that really stuck with me came from a woman I barely knew. She said she'd heard about my MS through mutual friends, and she wanted me to know that watching how I was handling it had inspired her to finally go to the doctor about some symptoms she'd been ignoring for months.

"If you can face MS head-on," she wrote, "I can face whatever this is too."

That message made me cry, but not from sadness. From joy. From the realization that God might be using my struggle to help other people find the courage to face their own struggles.

That's when I started to understand that my MS wasn't just happening to me—it was happening through me. It was giving me a platform, a voice, a story that could help other people who were dealing with their own health challenges, their own fears, their own moments of feeling like giving up.

People started coming to me for advice, for encouragement, for someone who understood what it felt like to have your life turned upside down by a medical diagnosis. They wanted to know how I stayed positive, how I managed my symptoms, how I dealt with the fear of the unknown.

I realized I had accidentally become something I never expected to be: an advocate, a voice of hope for people dealing with chronic illness.

The more I talked about my experience, the more I learned about how common these struggles really are. I met people with lupus, fibromyalgia, diabetes, depression, anxiety, autoimmune conditions I'd never heard of. I learned that millions of people are walking around carrying invisible battles, feeling alone in their struggles, afraid to speak up about what they're going through.

I also learned that most people don't know what to say to someone dealing with chronic illness. They either avoid the topic completely, offer empty platitudes like "everything happens for a reason," or share horror stories about people they knew who had the same condition.

None of those responses are helpful. What people really need is someone who will listen without judgment, someone who will acknowledge that their struggle is real without trying to minimize it or fix it, someone who will remind them that they're still the same valuable person they were before their diagnosis.

CHAPTER 13: FROM PAIN TO PURPOSE

I started to see that I could be that person for other people because I had been through it myself. I could offer something that healthy people, no matter how well-intentioned, couldn't offer: understanding from experience.

My friend Ty, who works in community health, approached me about speaking at a women's health program at my son's school. He said they needed someone to talk about living with chronic illness, and he thought I would be perfect for it.

My first instinct was to say no. I wasn't a professional speaker, wasn't an expert on anything except my own experience. Who was I to get up in front of people and give advice?

But then I thought about all the conversations I'd had with people who thanked me for being honest about my struggle, all the messages I'd received from people who said my story had helped them in some way. Maybe I didn't need to be an expert to be helpful. Maybe I just needed to be real.

"Let me think about it," I told him. But in my heart, I already knew I was going to say yes.

That speaking engagement hasn't happened yet, but I'm excited about it. Nervous, but excited. Because I know there will be women in that audience who are dealing with their own health challenges, their own fears, their own moments of wondering if they're strong enough to handle what life has thrown at them.

And I want to look them in the eye and tell them what someone needed to tell me in my darkest moments: You are stronger than you think you are. You have more fight in you than you realize. This challenge doesn't get to be the end of your story.

I want to tell them that having a chronic illness doesn't make you less valuable, less beautiful, less worthy of love and respect. It just makes you human in a way that's more visible than it is for people who haven't faced major health challenges yet.

I want to tell them that it's okay to grieve what you've lost while also celebrating what you still have. It's okay to have bad days and good days. It's okay to ask for help when you need it and to use whatever tools make your life easier.

Most importantly, I want to tell them that their struggle can become their strength, their pain can become their purpose, their test can become their testimony.

That's what happened to me. My MS, which felt like the worst thing that could ever happen to me, became the thing that gave my life new meaning, new direction, new purpose.

I'm not grateful for having MS—I wouldn't wish this condition on anyone. But I am grateful for what it taught me about myself, about resilience, about the power of community, about the importance of living each day fully because tomorrow isn't guaranteed.

I'm grateful that it connected me to a community of people I never would have met otherwise, people who understand struggles that healthy people can't understand.

I'm grateful that it gave me a story worth telling, a message worth sharing, a platform to help other people who are facing their own battles.

CHAPTER 13: FROM PAIN TO PURPOSE

My pain found its purpose. My struggle became my strength. My breakdown became my breakthrough.

And now, instead of asking "Why me?" I'm asking "What now? How can I use this experience to help someone else? What good can come from what felt like such a devastating loss?"

Those are much better questions to live with. Those are questions that lead to purpose instead of self-pity, to action instead of despair, to hope instead of hopelessness.

I don't know where this journey will take me next. Maybe I'll become a regular speaker at health events. Maybe I'll start a support group for people with chronic illnesses. Maybe I'll write articles or create resources or find other ways to share what I've learned.

What I do know is that my MS isn't just my burden anymore—it's also my gift. Not a gift I would have chosen, but a gift nonetheless. A gift that allows me to connect with people in a deep way, to offer hope to people who need it, to be living proof that you can face impossible things and not just survive them, but thrive in spite of them.

That's the purpose I found in my pain. That's the meaning I made from my struggle.

And that makes every hard day, every difficult moment, every challenge I've faced along the way worth it.

"Your pain always has the potential to become your purpose—you just have to be willing to share your story and let it help someone else write theirs." - E.N.

CHAPTER 14

THE SUPPORT SYSTEM THAT SAVED ME

I want to be real with you about something: I could not have done this alone.

The woman you're reading about, the one who got up from that bed and decided to fight, the one who refuses to let MS define her story—she didn't emerge in a vacuum. She was created by a community of people who refused to let her give up, who held her up when she couldn't hold herself up, who reminded her who she was when she forgot.

If you don't have a support system like that, I want you to know that you can build one. If you do have one, I want you to know how precious it is and how much you need to nurture it. Because the truth is, nobody fights chronic illness alone and wins. Nobody faces life-changing challenges in isolation and comes out stronger.

We need each other. We need people who will show up, speak truth, offer help, and refuse to let us disappear into our pain.

Let me tell you about the people who saved my life.

First, my doctor has been with me since day one of this journey, and I cannot overstate how important that relationship has been to my healing. She's not just my neurologist—she's my therapist, my cheerleader, my voice of reason, and sometimes my reality check all rolled into one.

From our very first appointment, she made me feel comfortable talking about what I was experiencing. She listened without judgment, answered my questions with patience, and most importantly, she saw me as a whole person, not just a collection of symptoms.

"You have MS," she told me early on, "but MS doesn't have you."

That became the foundation of everything that followed. She helped me understand that my diagnosis was something I was dealing with, not something I was becoming.

When I was going through my darkest period, when I was calling her office crying and desperate, she made time for me. She would spend an hour or more with me during appointments, letting me talk through my fears, my frustrations, my questions about the future.

"Everybody's body is different," she would remind me when I got scared by stories I heard or articles I read. "Don't listen to those stories. Your experience is going to be your experience, not someone else's."

She taught me to advocate for myself, to speak up when something wasn't working, to be an active participant in my treatment instead of a passive recipient. She encouraged me to ask questions, to do my own research, to take control of my health in every way I could.

CHAPTER 14: THE SUPPORT SYSTEM THAT SAVED ME

But more than that, she celebrated my victories with me. When my test results came back stable, when I had a good stretch of symptom-free days, when I accomplished something I wasn't sure I'd be able to do—she was genuinely happy for me, genuinely proud of how I was handling everything.

"You're doing great," she would tell me. "You're fine. I can see you doing what you're doing."

Having a doctor who believes in you, who sees your strength instead of just your limitations, who treats you like a partner instead of a patient—that makes all the difference in the world.

But my support system extended far beyond the medical community.

My family was my foundation. My mother-in-law, who sensed something was wrong that Sunday morning and sent her sister to check on me. My aunt-in-law, who prayed over me with the kind of authority that moves mountains. My brothers, who challenged me to keep fighting when I wanted to give up.

"You don't let that get to you," my brother would tell me when I called him crying. "You can do it. You can fight this. You've got kids to worry about, you know?"

He wasn't letting me wallow in self-pity. He was reminding me of my purpose, my reason for fighting. He was holding me accountable to be the woman he knew I was capable of being.

My friends were my lifeline to the world outside my diagnosis. They were the ones who kept inviting me to places even when I said no repeatedly. They were the ones who modified plans to accommodate my limitations without making me feel guilty about it. They were the ones who treated me like I was still me, not like I was fragile or broken or different.

One of my closest friends would do what she called "wellness checks" on me. She would call or text or just show up at my door to make sure I was okay, to make sure I wasn't isolating myself, to make sure I was still connected to life outside my apartment.

"Come on," she would say when I'd been in the house too long. "Let's go get something to eat. Let's go talk about it. You need to be out here with people."

She understood that being around people, seeing life happening, being part of community—that was medicine for me in a way that had nothing to do with pills or treatments.

My friends also gave me something I didn't know I needed: permission to still have fun. They showed me that having MS didn't mean my social life was over, didn't mean I couldn't enjoy myself, didn't mean I had to become someone who only talked about illness and symptoms and limitations.

When we would go out, they would make sure I had a place to sit if I needed it, make sure we didn't walk too far, make sure I felt included and comfortable. But they also expected me to laugh, to contribute to conversations, to be present and engaged. They struck the perfect balance between accommodation and expectation.

My support system also included people I didn't expect. Neighbors who would check on me, coworkers who would ask how I was doing, people from my community who would offer help or encouragement when they saw me struggling.

CHAPTER 14: THE SUPPORT SYSTEM THAT SAVED ME

There was one woman who saw me using my scooter and came up to me just to give me a hug. "I look up to you," she said. "You're so beautiful. You're doing it. I'm so proud of you."

That interaction lasted maybe two minutes, but it stayed with me for weeks. Sometimes support comes from the most unexpected places, from people who barely know you but see something in your struggle that speaks to their own experience.

I also found support online, in communities of people dealing with MS and other chronic illnesses. These were people who understood things that even my closest family and friends couldn't understand—the specific challenges of living with an unpredictable condition, the emotional toll of chronic illness, the frustration of dealing with invisible symptoms.

In these online spaces, I could talk about my worst days without feeling like I was burdening anyone. I could ask questions about symptoms or treatments without feeling embarrassed. I could celebrate small victories with people who understood why they were victories at all.

But here's what I learned about building and maintaining a support system: it requires honesty, vulnerability, and clear communication about what you need.

I had to learn to tell people what was helpful and what wasn't. I had to learn to say "I need you to listen right now, not try to fix anything" or "I need practical help with this specific thing" or "I need you to treat me normally, not like I'm sick."

I had to learn to accept help when it was offered, even when my pride wanted me to say I was fine. I had to learn that letting people help me wasn't a sign of weakness—it was a sign of wisdom, of understanding that we all need each other.

I also had to learn to set boundaries with people who weren't helpful, even if they meant well. The people who wanted to tell me horror stories about MS, who wanted to offer unsolicited medical advice, who wanted to treat me like I was dying—I had to learn to limit my exposure to that kind of energy.

"I appreciate your concern," I would say, "but what I need right now is positivity and encouragement, not scary stories or medical advice."

Building a support system also meant being part of other people's support systems in return. When my friends were going through difficult times, I showed up for them in whatever way I could. When other people in my MS communities were struggling, I offered encouragement and shared what had worked for me.

Support isn't a one-way street. It's a network of people taking care of each other, lifting each other up, sharing resources and hope and practical help.

The most important thing I learned about support systems is that you have to cultivate them before you need them. You can't wait until you're in crisis to start building relationships with people who care about you. You have to invest in community, in friendship, in family relationships when times are good so that foundation is there when times get hard.

I was lucky that I had already built strong relationships with family and friends before my diagnosis. But I also had to work to maintain those relationships and communicate with people about how my needs had changed.

If you're reading this and you don't feel like you have a strong support system, please know that it's never too late to start building one. Join a support group, connect with others who share your experiences, reach

CHAPTER 14: THE SUPPORT SYSTEM THAT SAVED ME

out to family members you've lost touch with, invest in friendships that matter to you.

And if you're reading this and you have people in your life who are dealing with chronic illness or other major challenges, please know that your support matters more than you realize. Your phone calls, your visits, your willingness to listen, your refusal to let them isolate themselves—all of that is literally life-saving.

We need each other. I needed my doctor, my family, my friends, my community, and even strangers who offered encouragement at just the right moment.

They saved my life by refusing to let me give up on it. They saved my spirit by reminding me who I was when I forgot. They saved my hope by holding onto it when I couldn't hold onto it myself.

That's what a support system does. That's why it's not optional. That's why building and maintaining community isn't just nice to have—it's essential for survival, for healing, for thriving in the face of whatever challenges life throws at you.

I am who I am today because of the people who surrounded me, supported me, and refused to let me disappear into my pain.

And I hope that I can be that kind of support for someone else who needs it.

"A support system isn't just people who are there when you fall—it's people who remind you how to get back up, and who celebrate with you when you do." - E.N.

CHAPTER 15

LIVE. DON'T CLAIM IT.

"**I**t's a minor thing."

That's what I tell people when they ask me about my MS. Not because it's actually minor—having a chronic, unpredictable autoimmune disease that affects your nervous system is definitely not minor. But because calling it minor in my own mind helps me keep it in perspective. It helps me remember that this is one part of my life, not the whole thing.

"Don't claim it."

That's what I tell people when they start identifying too closely with their diagnosis, when they start introducing themselves by their illness, when they start letting their condition become their entire identity.

These two phrases have become my life philosophy, my way of staying mentally and emotionally healthy while dealing with something that could easily consume my entire existence if I let it.

Let me explain what I mean by "don't claim it," because it's not about denial or pretending your condition doesn't exist. It's about refusing to let your diagnosis become your identity.

There's a difference between saying "I have MS" and saying "I am an MS patient." There's a difference between acknowledging that you're dealing with something challenging and making that challenge the center of your universe. There's a difference between managing a condition and letting that condition manage you.

When you claim an illness, you give it power over your entire life. You start seeing everything through the lens of that diagnosis. You start making decisions based on fear of what might happen instead of hope for what could happen. You start limiting yourself before your condition even limits you.

I see people do this all the time. They get a diagnosis, and suddenly that's all they talk about, all they think about, all they research, all they plan around. They join every support group, read every article, follow every social media account related to their condition. They become experts on their illness but forget to be experts on their own life.

That's claiming it. And I refuse to do it.

Instead, I acknowledge that I have MS, I take it seriously, I manage it responsibly, I educate myself about it, I take my medications, I go to my appointments, I make necessary accommodations. But I don't let it define who I am or limit what I believe is possible for my life.

I have MS, but I am Eunice Newton. I am Tweety from Harlem. I am a mother, a friend, a community member, a woman with dreams and goals and things I want to accomplish. MS is just one thing I have to factor in as I pursue all of those other aspects of my identity.

CHAPTER 15: LIVE. DON'T CLAIM IT.

The "minor thing" part of my philosophy is about perspective. Yes, MS is serious. Yes, it affects my daily life. Yes, it requires ongoing management and attention. But in the grand scheme of my existence, in the context of all the other things that matter to me, it's a minor thing.

My relationship with my children? That's a major thing. My faith? That's a major thing. My friendships, my community connections, my purpose in life? Those are major things. MS is just something I have to work around as I focus on those major things.

This mindset shift changes everything. Instead of waking up every morning thinking about MS, I wake up thinking about what I want to accomplish that day. Instead of planning my life around my limitations, I plan my life around my priorities and then figure out how to work around any limitations.

Instead of seeing myself as someone who is sick, I see myself as someone who is living—fully, intentionally, joyfully—despite dealing with a health challenge.

This philosophy extends beyond just chronic illness. It applies to any challenge, any setback, any difficulty you might face in life.

Don't claim your depression—acknowledge it, treat it, manage it, but don't let it become your entire identity. Don't claim your financial struggles—work on them, learn from them, but don't let them define your worth or limit your dreams. Don't claim your relationship problems, your family dysfunction, your past trauma—deal with these things, get help for them, heal from them, but don't let them become the central story of your life.

You are so much more than the worst thing that has happened to you. You are so much more than your biggest challenge. You are so much more than your diagnosis, your struggle, your setback.

Live. Don't claim it.

Live like you're a whole person dealing with a challenge, not like you're a challenge that happens to be attached to a person. Live like your condition is something you're managing, not something that's managing you. Live like you have a future worth planning for, dreams worth pursuing, goals worth working toward.

This doesn't mean ignoring reality or being recklessly optimistic. It means being realistic about your challenges while refusing to let those challenges become your ceiling.

I'm realistic about my MS. I know I have good days and bad days. I know I need to pace myself differently than I used to. I know I need to be careful about stress and heat and overexertion. I know I need to take my medications and keep my appointments and monitor my symptoms.

But I'm also realistic about my capabilities, my strength, my resilience, my ability to adapt and overcome and find ways to live fully despite this diagnosis.

I'm realistic about the fact that I might have this condition for the rest of my life, but I'm also realistic about the fact that I can have a beautiful, meaningful, impactful life with this condition.

The key is not letting fear of what might happen keep you from living what's happening right now.

CHAPTER 15: LIVE. DON'T CLAIM IT.

I could spend all my time worrying about whether my MS will get worse, whether I'll end up in a wheelchair, whether I'll be able to take care of myself as I get older. And you know what? That worry wouldn't prevent any of those things from happening if they're going to happen. But that worry would definitely prevent me from enjoying the good health I have right now, the mobility I have right now, the capabilities I have right now.

So I choose to focus on now. I choose to live fully in this moment, with this body, with these capabilities, with this life. I'll deal with whatever comes next when it comes, but I'm not going to sacrifice today's joy for tomorrow's potential problems.

That's what "live, don't claim it" means to me. It means choosing life over fear, hope over despair, possibility over limitation.

It means eating good food because it nourishes my body and brings me joy, not because I'm trying to cure my MS through diet. It means exercising because it makes me feel strong and capable, not because I'm trying to prevent progression of my symptoms. It means spending time with friends because I love them and they make me laugh, not because social connection is supposed to be good for people with chronic illnesses.

I do things because I want to do them, because they add value to my life, because they align with my priorities and goals. The fact that some of these things might also be good for managing my MS is a bonus, not the primary motivation.

This mindset has allowed me to live a full, rich life over the past five years since my diagnosis. I've traveled, I've maintained my friendships, I've been present for my children, I've found new purpose in sharing my story, I've continued to be an active member of my community.

None of that would have been possible if I had claimed MS as my identity, if I had let it become the center of my universe, if I had started seeing myself primarily as a sick person trying to get by rather than as a whole person living fully.

Your diagnosis, whatever it is, doesn't get to write your story. Your circumstances, however challenging, don't get to determine your identity. Your limitations, however real, don't get to define your possibilities.

You get to decide how to respond to what happens to you. You get to decide what story to tell about your life. You get to decide whether to focus on what you can't do or what you can do, what you've lost or what you still have, what might go wrong or what could go right.

I decided to live. Not just survive, not just get by, not just make it through each day, but really live. Live with intention, with joy, with purpose, with hope.

I decided not to claim MS as my identity but to claim strength, resilience, faith, love, community, purpose—all the things that make life worth living regardless of what challenges you're facing.

That decision has made all the difference.

Live. Don't claim it.

Whatever "it" is for you—chronic illness, mental health struggles, financial difficulties, relationship problems, family dysfunction, past trauma, current crisis—don't let it become bigger than your entire life.

Acknowledge it. Deal with it. Get help for it. Learn from it. But don't claim it as your identity.

CHAPTER 15: LIVE. DON'T CLAIM IT.

Instead, claim your strength. Claim your resilience. Claim your capacity for joy, for love, for growth, for contribution, for making a difference in the world.

Claim your life. And then live it.

"The difference between surviving and thriving isn't about what happens to you—it's about how much power you give those circumstances over your identity and your future." - E.N.

PART VI: MESSAGES FOR WARRIORS

CHAPTER 16

YOU CAN GET UP TOO

Beautiful, I'm talking to you.

Yeah, you—the one who picked up this book because something in your life has knocked you down and you're wondering if you have what it takes to get back up. The one who's lying in your own version of that bed I was stuck in, staring at your own ceiling, wondering if this is just how life is going to be from now on.

The one who's tired of being tired, scared of being scared, stuck in your own story of limitation and loss and "what if I can't handle this?"

I want you to listen to me very carefully: You can get up too.

I'm not saying it because it sounds nice or because it's what you want to hear. I'm saying it because I know it's true. I know it's true because I've been where you are, and I've seen what's possible when you make the decision to fight for your life instead of just existing in it.

I know it's true because I've watched my daughter get up from academic failure and fight for the grades she wanted. I've watched my community members get up from their own health scares and take control of their wellness. I've watched strangers reach out to me after hearing my story and find the courage to face their own diagnoses, their own fears, their own challenges.

I know it's true because getting up isn't about being superhuman or having some special strength that other people don't have. Getting up is about remembering that you have a choice in how you respond to what happens to you.

And right now, you have a choice to make.

You can stay where you are—in that bed, in that mindset, in that story that says you're too weak, too sick, too broken, too overwhelmed to handle what life has thrown at you. You can keep telling yourself that other people are stronger than you, that other people have better support systems than you, that other people have easier challenges than you.

Or you can decide that today is the day you start getting up.

Not all at once. Not perfectly. Not without setbacks or bad days or moments when you want to crawl back under those covers and hide from the world.

But piece by piece, day by day, choice by choice, you can start the process of reclaiming your life from whatever has been holding you down.

Let me tell you what getting up looks like, because it's probably not what you think.

Getting up doesn't mean pretending everything is fine. It doesn't mean putting on a brave face and acting like you're not struggling. It doesn't mean being positive all the time or never having moments of fear or sadness or anger about your situation.

Getting up means acknowledging where you are while refusing to stay there. It means feeling your feelings while also taking action to change your circumstances. It means being honest about your limitations while also being creative about your possibilities.

Getting up means asking for help when you need it. It means using whatever tools, accommodations, or support systems you need to function. It means letting people love you even when you don't feel lovable, letting people help you even when your pride wants you to handle everything alone.

Getting up means taking care of your body in whatever way you can—eating food that nourishes you, moving in ways that feel good, resting when you need to rest, getting medical care when you need medical care. It means treating your body like the precious vessel it is, not like an enemy that's betraying you.

Getting up means taking care of your mind and your spirit too. It means finding sources of joy, beauty, connection, and meaning even in the middle of difficult circumstances. It means protecting your mental and emotional energy by limiting exposure to things and people that drain you, and increasing exposure to things and people that fill you up.

Getting up means being selective about the stories you tell yourself and the stories you let other people tell you about your situation. It means challenging thoughts that limit you unnecessarily and embracing thoughts that remind you of your strength, your worth, your potential.

Getting up means focusing on what you can control instead of what you can't control. You can't control your diagnosis, but you can control how you manage it. You can't control other people's reactions to your situation, but you can control who you choose to share it with. You can't control what happened to you, but you can control what you do next.

Getting up means remembering that you are not your circumstances. You are not your diagnosis, your trauma, your loss, your setback, your struggle. You are a whole person who happens to be dealing with challenging circumstances. You are someone with a history of overcoming things, even if you don't remember that right now.

Getting up means connecting with your purpose, your reason for fighting. For me, it was my kids—I couldn't let them watch their mama give up. For you, it might be your children, your partner, your parents, your friends, your career, your dreams, your community, your faith, or simply your own belief that you deserve to live a full and beautiful life.

Getting up means taking it one day at a time, one moment at a time, one choice at a time. You don't have to figure out the rest of your life right now. You just have to figure out the next right thing to do, and then do it.

Maybe the next right thing is getting out of bed. Maybe it's taking a shower. Maybe it's making a phone call to someone who cares about you. Maybe it's scheduling a doctor's appointment you've been putting off. Maybe it's eating something nourishing. Maybe it's going outside for five minutes. Maybe it's writing in a journal. Maybe it's listening to music that lifts your spirit.

The next right thing doesn't have to be big or dramatic or life-changing. It just has to be one small step in the direction of taking care of yourself, of reclaiming your agency, of choosing life over despair.

And then, after you do that one small thing, you do the next small thing. And then the next. And slowly, gradually, those small things add up to big changes, big shifts, big transformations.

That's how I got up. Not in one heroic moment, but in a thousand small moments where I chose to keep going instead of giving up, where I chose to try instead of surrendering, where I chose to believe in possibility instead of accepting limitation.

I want you to know that the voice that told me I could do it—that voice is available to you too. It might sound like a loved one who has passed away, or a family member who believes in you, or God speaking directly to your heart, or your own inner wisdom that knows you're stronger than your circumstances.

Listen for that voice. Trust that voice. And when you hear it, do what it says.

Get up.

Not because it's easy—it's not easy. Not because you feel ready—you might never feel ready. Not because you have all the answers—none of us have all the answers.

Get up because you deserve to live, not just exist. Get up because the world needs what you have to offer. Get up because your story isn't over yet, and the best chapters might still be ahead of you.

Get up because every time someone gets up, it makes it easier for the next person to get up too. Your recovery, your resilience, your refusal to stay down—that becomes part of the collective story of human strength that helps other people believe they can be strong too.

I got up for my kids, for my family, for my community, for myself. But I also got up for you—for the person I didn't know yet who would read this book and need to know that getting up is possible, that recovery is possible, that thriving in the face of challenges is possible.

You can get up too. Not because I'm special or because I had some advantage you don't have, but because the capacity for resilience, for healing, for transformation lives inside every human being. It lives inside you, even if it's buried under pain and fear and exhaustion right now.

It's there. It's waiting. It's ready.

All you have to do is make the choice.

Get up, beautiful. Your life is waiting for you.

The world is waiting for you.

I'm waiting for you.

And that voice inside you that knows you can do it? It's waiting too.

Listen to it. Trust it. Follow it.

Get up.

You can do it.

I believe in you.

"The moment you decide to get up is the moment you remember that you've always had the power to choose your response to life's challenges. That power never left you—it was just waiting for you to use it again." - E.N.

CHAPTER 17

TAKE CARE OF YOURSELF

If I could give you just one piece of advice—one thing that could change your life regardless of what challenge you're facing—it would be this: take care of yourself.

I know that sounds simple, maybe even obvious. But let me tell you, most of us are walking around not taking care of ourselves, and we don't even realize it. We're so busy taking care of everyone else, so focused on meeting external demands, so convinced that self-care is selfish, that we ignore our bodies, neglect our emotional needs, and wonder why we feel exhausted, overwhelmed, and susceptible to whatever life throws at us.

Before my MS diagnosis, I thought I was taking care of myself. I was working, paying bills, raising my kids, showing up for my family and friends. I thought being tired at the end of every day meant I was living life right, that pushing through discomfort was a sign of strength, that ignoring my body's signals was what responsible adults did.

I was wrong about all of that.

The truth is, I was running myself into the ground. I was eating fast food more often than home-cooked meals. I was staying up too late because that was the only time I had to myself. I was ignoring symptoms because I didn't have time to be sick. I was treating my body like a machine that was supposed to keep running no matter what I put it through.

And then my body said, "We need to talk."

MS forced me to learn how to take care of myself, and that learning process probably saved my life in more ways than one. Not just from the specific effects of my autoimmune condition, but from the general effects of living in a way that wasn't sustainable, wasn't healthy, wasn't honoring the fact that I only get one body and one life.

So let me share with you what I learned about taking care of yourself, because whether you're dealing with a chronic illness or just trying to live your best life, these lessons apply.

First, and most importantly: food is medicine.

I cannot emphasize this enough. What you put in your body matters more than you probably realize. It affects your energy, your mood, your immune system, your ability to think clearly, your capacity to handle stress, your sleep quality—everything.

Before my diagnosis, I was eating whatever was convenient, whatever was fast, whatever the kids wanted. McDonald's, Chinese takeout, processed foods, sugary drinks—if it was quick and easy, that's what I was putting in my body.

CHAPTER 17: TAKE CARE OF YOURSELF

But my doctor opened my eyes to something important: "It's in the food," she told me. "A lot of these conditions we're seeing, we don't even know where they're coming from, but it's in the food."

That conversation changed how I think about eating. I realized that every time I eat something, I'm either feeding health or feeding illness. I'm either giving my body what it needs to function optimally, or I'm giving it substances that make it harder for my immune system, my nervous system, my digestive system to do their jobs.

Now I cook at home most of the time. I read labels. I choose fresh ingredients over processed ones. I drink water—lots and lots of water—instead of juice or soda. When I want Chinese food, I look up how to make it at home instead of ordering it from a restaurant where I don't know what's in it or how it's prepared.

This doesn't mean I never eat anything fun or that I've become obsessive about food. It means I'm intentional about what I put in my body most of the time, and when I do eat something that's not the healthiest choice, I do it mindfully rather than mindlessly.

The difference in how I feel is incredible. My energy is more stable, my mood is more consistent, and I genuinely believe that eating better has helped me manage my MS symptoms more effectively.

Second: move your body in ways that feel good.

I used to think exercise meant going to the gym and doing workouts I hated. I thought it had to be intense and time-consuming to count. I thought if I wasn't sweating and miserable, I wasn't doing it right.

Now I understand that movement is about taking care of your body, not punishing it. It's about maintaining strength, flexibility, and cardiovascular health so you can do the things that matter to you.

For me, that means physical therapy twice a week to help with my MS symptoms. It means walking when I can, using my scooter when I need to, and not feeling guilty about either choice. It means stretching, dancing (even if it's just swaying to music while sitting down), and finding ways to keep my body active within my current capabilities.

The key is consistency, not intensity. A little bit of movement every day is better than intense workouts that you can't maintain. Find what feels good to your body and do that, regularly.

Third: your mental and emotional health are just as important as your physical health.

This was the hardest lesson for me to learn, because I was raised in a generation and a community where mental health wasn't talked about much. You were supposed to be strong, push through, handle your problems on your own.

But dealing with a chronic illness taught me that you can't separate your mental and emotional wellbeing from your physical wellbeing. Stress can trigger flares. Depression can make symptoms worse. Anxiety can interfere with healing.

Taking care of your mental health might mean therapy, medication, support groups, meditation, prayer, journaling, or whatever helps you process your emotions in healthy ways. It means setting boundaries with people who drain your energy. It means saying no to commitments that overwhelm you. It means asking for help when you need it.

CHAPTER 17: TAKE CARE OF YOURSELF

For me, music is medicine for my mental health. When I put on my headphones and listen to songs that lift my spirit, I can literally feel my stress level decrease. Prayer and my faith community provide emotional support that keeps me grounded. Talking to friends who understand my situation helps me feel less alone.

Fourth: sleep is not optional.

I used to think staying up late was giving me more time to get things done. I used to wear my ability to function on little sleep like a badge of honor.

Now I understand that sleep is when your body repairs itself, when your immune system does its most important work, when your brain processes the day's experiences and prepares for tomorrow's challenges.

I prioritize getting enough sleep now, even if it means some things don't get done. I've learned that I'm more productive, more patient, more emotionally stable, and physically stronger when I'm well-rested.

Fifth: go to the doctor.

This should be obvious, but so many people avoid medical care until they're in crisis. They ignore symptoms, put off appointments, hope problems will resolve themselves.

Don't do that. Your body is the only one you get. Take it seriously. Get regular checkups. Address problems when they're small instead of waiting until they're big. Be an advocate for yourself in medical settings—ask questions, get second opinions if you need them, make sure you understand your treatment options.

If you don't have health insurance or access to regular medical care, look for community health centers, free clinics, or other resources in your area. Your health is worth the effort it takes to find care.

Sixth: create a support system and use it.

Taking care of yourself includes recognizing that you can't do everything alone. You need people who care about you, who will check on you, who will help you when you need help, who will celebrate with you when things go well.

This might mean strengthening relationships with family and friends, joining support groups, connecting with neighbors, or finding community through shared interests or values.

And when people offer help, say yes. When people ask how you're doing, be honest. When you need something, ask for it. This isn't being needy or weak—this is being human.

Finally: be gentle with yourself.

Taking care of yourself means treating yourself with the same kindness and compassion you would show to someone you love. It means understanding that you're going to have good days and bad days, that healing isn't linear, that setbacks don't mean failure.

It means celebrating small victories, forgiving yourself for mistakes, and remembering that you're doing the best you can with the resources you have right now.

Taking care of yourself isn't selfish—it's necessary. You can't pour from an empty cup. You can't take care of other people if you don't take care of yourself first. You can't handle life's challenges if you're running on empty physically, emotionally, and spiritually.

CHAPTER 17: TAKE CARE OF YOURSELF

The airline safety instruction applies to life too: put on your own oxygen mask first, then help others with theirs.

Whether you're dealing with a health crisis, a family emergency, work stress, financial problems, or just the general demands of daily life, the foundation for handling all of it is taking care of yourself.

Your body, your mind, your spirit—they're all you've got. Treat them well. Nourish them. Protect them. Honor them.

You deserve to be healthy. You deserve to be strong. You deserve to be well-rested, well-fed, emotionally supported, and physically capable of doing the things that matter to you.

But you're the only one who can make that happen. You're the only one who can choose to prioritize your own wellbeing. You're the only one who can make the daily decisions that add up to a life of health and vitality.

So please, beautiful—take care of yourself. Not tomorrow, not next week, not when things calm down or when you have more time or when other people don't need you as much.

Start today. Start right now.

Your future self will thank you.

"Taking care of yourself isn't preparation for your real life—it is your real life. Every choice you make to nourish your body, mind, and spirit is a choice to honor the gift of being alive." - E.N.

CHAPTER 18

LETTER FROM EUNICE

My Dear Beautiful Warrior,

I'm sitting here in my kitchen in Harlem, five years after that terrifying night when I first heard the words "Multiple Sclerosis," and I want to tell you something: I made it. Not just survived—I made it to a place where I can honestly say I'm thriving.

I'm writing this letter to you because I know you're out there. You're the person who picked up this book because something in your life has knocked you down and you're wondering if you have what it takes to get back up. You're the person lying in your own version of that bed I was stuck in, staring at your own ceiling, wondering if this is just how life is going to be from now on.

You're the person who feels broken, scared, overwhelmed, and maybe even hopeless about whatever challenge you're facing. You might be dealing with a health diagnosis like mine, or depression, or loss, or trauma, or financial struggles, or family problems, or any of the thousand things that can make life feel impossible to navigate.

I want you to know that I see you. I understand you. I've been you.

And I want you to know that your story isn't over.

Five years ago, I thought my life was finished. I thought the woman I had been—the one who never sat still, who took care of everyone, who was known for her strength and resilience—was gone forever. I thought MS had stolen not just my health, but my identity, my future, my reason for being.

I was wrong about all of that.

The woman I am today is stronger than the woman I was before my diagnosis. Not physically—my body will never be what it once was. But emotionally, spiritually, mentally, I am more resilient, more grateful, more intentional, more aware of what really matters than I ever was when I thought I was invincible.

I've learned things about myself, about life, about love, about community, about faith that I never would have learned if everything had stayed easy. I've discovered reserves of strength I didn't know I had. I've built relationships deeper than any I had before. I've found purpose in my pain and meaning in my struggle.

I've become someone I'm proud to be, someone my children can look up to, someone my community can count on, someone who can offer hope to other people who are facing their own battles.

That didn't happen overnight. It didn't happen without setbacks, without bad days, without moments when I wanted to give up all over again. Healing isn't linear, and neither is growth. There were days when I felt like I was back at square one, when I questioned whether I was really as strong as people said I was.

CHAPTER 18: LETTER FROM EUNICE

But I kept getting up. Every time life knocked me down, I found a way to get back up. Not because I was special or because I had some advantage you don't have, but because I made a choice—over and over again, day after day—to fight for my life instead of just existing in it.

You have that same choice available to you right now.

I know it doesn't feel like it. When you're in the middle of a crisis, when you're overwhelmed by circumstances you never asked for, when you're dealing with challenges that feel bigger than your capacity to handle them, choice can feel like a luxury you can't afford.

But choice is the one thing that can never be taken away from you. You might not be able to choose what happens to you, but you can always choose how you respond to what happens to you.

You can choose to ask for help instead of suffering in silence. You can choose to take care of your body instead of ignoring its needs. You can choose to speak kindly to yourself instead of beating yourself up for not being perfect. You can choose to focus on what you can control instead of what you can't control.

You can choose to believe that your current circumstances are temporary instead of permanent. You can choose to look for possibilities instead of only seeing limitations. You can choose to treat yourself with compassion instead of criticism.

Most importantly, you can choose to keep going. One day at a time, one moment at a time, one breath at a time if that's all you can manage.

I want you to know that you're not alone in this fight. There are people who care about you, even if you can't see them right now. There are resources available to help you, even if you haven't found them yet. There is hope for your situation, even if you can't feel it right now.

I want you to know that asking for help isn't a sign of weakness—it's a sign of wisdom. Using tools and accommodations that make your life easier isn't giving up—it's being smart. Having bad days doesn't mean you're failing—it means you're human.

I want you to know that you don't have to be perfect to be valuable. You don't have to have it all figured out to be worthy of love and support. You don't have to be strong every moment of every day to be considered strong.

I want you to know that your struggle is not your identity. Whatever you're going through—illness, loss, trauma, setback—that's something you're dealing with, not something you are. You are so much more than your circumstances, so much more than your worst days, so much more than your biggest challenges.

You are a whole person with a history of overcoming things, with people who care about you, with gifts to offer the world, with a future worth fighting for.

I want you to know that it's okay to grieve what you've lost while also celebrating what you still have. It's okay to acknowledge that things are hard while also believing they can get better. It's okay to be realistic about your limitations while also being hopeful about your possibilities.

I want you to know that healing happens. Recovery happens. Transformation happens. Not always in the ways we expect or on the timeline we want, but it happens. I've seen it in my own life and in the lives of

CHAPTER 18: LETTER FROM EUNICE

countless other people who refused to let their circumstances have the final word.

I want you to know that your story matters. Your experience, your perspective, your journey through whatever you're facing—all of that has value, not just to you but to other people who need to see that it's possible to face hard things and come out stronger.

Someday, when you're on the other side of this challenge, someone else is going to need to hear your story. Someone else is going to need to see proof that people can face what you're facing and not just survive, but thrive.

You might become someone else's hope, someone else's inspiration, someone else's evidence that getting up is possible.

But first, you have to get up yourself.

I'm not going to lie to you and tell you it's going to be easy. It's not easy. Some days are going to be harder than others. Some setbacks are going to knock you down again just when you thought you were making progress.

But I am going to tell you that it's worth it. The life that's waiting for you on the other side of this struggle—the strength you'll discover, the relationships you'll build, the purpose you'll find, the joy you'll experience—all of that is worth fighting for.

You are worth fighting for.

So please, beautiful—don't give up. Not today, not tomorrow, not ever. Keep looking for the light, even when the darkness feels overwhelming. Keep reaching for help, even when you feel like a burden. Keep believing in possibilities, even when the present feels impossible.

Listen for that voice that tells you "you can do it"—the voice that sounds like love, like strength, like everything in you that refuses to be defeated. Trust that voice. Follow that voice. Let that voice guide you back to life, back to hope, back to the person you're meant to become through all of this.

Your story isn't over. The best chapters might still be ahead of you. The person you're becoming through this struggle might be exactly who the world needs you to be.

I believe in you. I'm rooting for you. I'm here in Harlem, living proof that people can face impossible things and not just survive them, but find joy, purpose, and meaning in the middle of them.

You can do it too. I know you can.

Now get up, beautiful. Your life is waiting for you.

With all my love and all my faith in your strength,

Eunice "Tweety" Newton

P.S. Remember: It's a minor thing. Don't claim it. Live your life. Take care of yourself. And never, ever give up.

You've got this.

"Every ending is also a beginning. Every breakdown can become a breakthrough. Every time you get up, you prove to yourself and to the world that the human spirit is stronger than any circumstance." - E.N.

ACKNOWLEDGMENTS

When I think about everyone who helped make this book possible, I get overwhelmed with gratitude. This story didn't happen in isolation, and this book couldn't have been written without a community of people who believed in me, supported me, and refused to let me give up.

First and foremost, I want to thank God for giving me the strength to get through the darkest days and the wisdom to find purpose in my pain. My faith has been the foundation of everything—my healing, my hope, and my ability to share this story with others who need to hear it.

To my children—my heart, my motivation, my reason for fighting every single day. You watched your mama go through something scary and difficult, and instead of losing faith in me, you became my biggest cheerleaders. To my son, who keeps me moving with his basketball games and his beautiful spirit. To my daughters, who challenge me to be strong and celebrate every victory with me. You are my pulse, my purpose, and my greatest accomplishment. Everything I do is for you.

To my man, my partner of over 23 years and the father of my three beautiful children—thank you for being there through it all. You never treated me like I was broken, you stepped up when I needed you to step up, and you've shown our kids what it means to stand by someone through thick and thin. You take our son to basketball practice when I can't, you help when I need help, and you've never made me feel like a burden. Your quiet strength has been one of my anchors through this storm.

To my mother-in-law, who knew something was wrong before I even admitted it to myself, and who sent help exactly when I needed it. Your intuition and your love saved my life. To my aunt-in-law, who prayed over me with the kind of power that moves mountains and reminded me that I was going to be alright. Your prayer broke chains I didn't even know were holding me down.

To my brothers, who wouldn't let me feel sorry for myself, who challenged me to keep fighting, who reminded me that I had kids to live for when I wanted to give up. Your tough love was exactly what I needed, exactly when I needed it.

To my entire family—the ones who called to check on me, who came to visit, who held me up when I couldn't hold myself up, who never treated me like I was fragile or broken, who expected me to keep being the strong woman they'd always known. Your expectations helped me live up to them.

To my cousin, who is no longer here but whose words still guide me every day. The text message you sent me before you passed away, telling me you looked up to me, became one of my greatest motivations to keep fighting. I'm telling my story for both of us—for me and for you, who couldn't tell yours. I love you and I miss you.

To my doctor, Dr. Sylvia Klineova, my neurologist, who has been so much more than a doctor to me. You've been my therapist, my cheerleader, my voice of reason, and my source of hope. You taught me that I have MS, but MS doesn't have me. You celebrated every victory with me and held space for every fear. You made me feel comfortable in my new body and confident about my future. Thank you for seeing me as a whole person, not just a collection of symptoms.

To my close friends, who did wellness checks on me, who wouldn't let me disappear into my diagnosis, who kept inviting me places even when I said no, who modified plans to include me without making me feel guilty about my limitations. You kept me connected to life outside of MS, and that connection probably saved my sanity.

To all my friends who treated me like I was still me—who expected me to laugh, to contribute to conversations, to be present and engaged, who struck the perfect balance between accommodation and expectation. You showed me that having MS didn't mean I couldn't still have fun, still enjoy life, still be the person you'd always known me to be.

To my community in Harlem, who embraced me when I finally got the courage to be open about my diagnosis. You didn't treat me like I was broken or tragic. You asked thoughtful questions, shared your own struggles, and made me feel like my honesty was a gift, not a burden. You taught me that vulnerability can be a fotrm of service.

To everyone who reached out to me after hearing about my MS—the old friends, the acquaintances, the people I barely knew who took the time to send messages of support and encouragement. Your words came at moments when I needed them most, and they reminded me that I wasn't alone in this fight.

To the online community of people living with MS and other chronic illnesses, who understood things that even my closest family and friends couldn't understand. You gave me space to talk about my worst days without feeling like a burden, and you celebrated my victories with people who truly understood why they were victories.

To Ty, who saw something in me that I didn't see in myself and asked me to speak at the women's health program. You gave me my first opportunity to turn my pain into purpose, to use my story to help other people. That invitation changed how I see myself and my role in the community.

To everyone who will read this book and find hope, encouragement, or practical guidance in these pages—thank you for giving my story purpose. Thank you for proving that our struggles don't have to be meaningless, that our pain can become someone else's healing, that our tests can become our testimonies.

To Makeda James, who conducted the interviews that became the foundation of this book. You created a safe space for me to share my story, asked the right questions to draw out the important details, and helped me see that what I'd been through was worth sharing with the world. Your skill as an interviewer and your compassion as a human being made this book possible.

To my childhood friend and publisher Ash Cash Exantus, who believed in my story from the very beginning and made this dream a reality. Your friendship has spanned decades, and now you've helped me turn my pain into purpose by bringing this book to life. Thank you for seeing the value in my journey and for having the vision to know that others needed to hear it.

To my writing team at 1Brick Publishing, who took my spoken words and helped shape them into something that could reach people beyond my immediate community. Thank you for honoring my voice while helping me craft it into something that could inspire and encourage others.

To everyone who has supported me in ways big and small—the people who gave me rides when I couldn't drive, who brought food when I was too tired to cook, who listened when I needed to talk, who celebrated when I had good news, who simply showed up when showing up mattered.

To my boss, who noticed I was limping and told me to go to the hospital. Your observation probably saved my life, or at least saved me from suffering longer than I had to. Sometimes the people who care about us see things we can't see ourselves.

To every healthcare worker, therapist, and medical professional who has been part of my journey. You do important work that makes it possible for people like me to not just survive our diagnoses, but thrive with them.

To everyone who is living with MS, chronic illness, or any other challenge that makes life more complicated—thank you for showing me what courage looks like every single day. You inspire me to keep fighting, keep growing, keep believing that we can live full, beautiful lives regardless of our circumstances.

And finally, to anyone who reads this book and finds the strength to get up from whatever has knocked them down—you are the reason this story needed to be told. You are the reason I had to get up first. Your healing, your recovery, your refusal to give up is what makes all of this meaningful.

This book exists because a community of people refused to let me disappear into my diagnosis. I pray that it will help create communities for other people who need the same kind of support, the same kind of hope, the same reminder that they are stronger than their circumstances.

We all need each other. We all need reminders that we can do hard things. We all need proof that getting up is possible.

Thank you for being part of my story. Thank you for letting me be part of yours.

With endless gratitude and love,

Eunice "Tweety" Newton

RESOURCES FOR MS AWARENESS AND SUPPORT

If you or someone you love is dealing with Multiple Sclerosis, please know that you are not alone. There are many organizations, resources, and communities dedicated to supporting people with MS and their families. Here are some places to start:

National Organizations

National Multiple Sclerosis Society

- Website: nationalmssociety.org
- Phone: 1-800-344-4867
- Services: Information, support groups, financial assistance, advocacy, research funding
- Local chapters available nationwide

Multiple Sclerosis Association of America (MSAA)

- Website: mymsaa.org
- Phone: 1-800-532-7667

- Services: Equipment distribution, cooling products, MRI funding, educational resources

Multiple Sclerosis Foundation

- Website: msfocus.org
- Phone: 1-888-673-6287
- Services: Support services, educational programs, publications

Online Support Communities

MyMSTeam

- Website: myMSteam.com
- The social network for people living with multiple sclerosis

MS Views and News

- Website: msviewsandnews.org
- Educational resources and community support

Multiple Sclerosis News Today

- Website: multiplesclerosisnewstoday.com
- Latest news, research updates, and patient stories

Financial and Practical Support

MS Lifelines

- Phone: 1-877-447-3243
- Patient support program offering financial assistance and resources

Chronic Disease Fund

- Website: cdfund.org
- Financial assistance for medication copays

Patient Advocate Foundation

- Website: patientadvocate.org
- Phone: 1-800-532-5274
- Help with insurance, financial, and employment issues

Educational Resources

Can Do Multiple Sclerosis

- Website: cando-ms.org
- Wellness and lifestyle programs for people with MS

MS Learning Channel

- Website: mslearningchannel.com
- Educational webinars and resources

For Families and Caregivers

Well Spouse Association

- Website: wellspouse.org
- Support for spouses and partners of chronically ill individuals

National Family Caregivers Association

- Website: caregiving.org

- Resources and support for family caregivers

Emergency Resources

National Suicide Prevention Lifeline

- Phone: 988
- 24/7 crisis support for anyone experiencing suicidal thoughts

Crisis Text Line

- Text HOME to 741741
- 24/7 crisis support via text message

Important Notes

- Always consult with qualified healthcare professionals for medical advice
- These resources are provided for informational purposes and do not constitute medical recommendations
- Contact information may change; please verify current details on organization websites
- If you're in crisis, please reach out for help immediately

Remember Eunice's Words

"You don't have to face this alone. There are people who understand what you're going through, resources to help you navigate this journey, and hope for living a full, meaningful life with MS. Take it one day at a time, ask for help when you need it, and never give up on yourself."

ABOUT THE AUTHOR

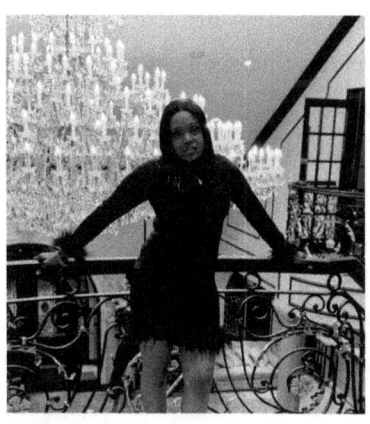

Eunice "Tweety" Newton is a mother, advocate, and inspirational speaker from Harlem, New York. Diagnosed with Multiple Sclerosis in 2019 at the age of 36, Eunice transformed her personal struggle into a mission of hope and encouragement for others facing life's most challenging moments.

Before her diagnosis, Eunice worked as a teaching assistant, dedicating herself to supporting children's education and development. Known throughout her community for her vibrant personality and unwavering strength, she was always the person others could count on—the friend who showed up, the family member who offered support, the community member who made a difference.

When MS entered her life, Eunice faced a period of profound depression and uncertainty. But with the support of her faith, her three children, her medical team, and her Harlem community, she discovered an inner strength that not only helped her rebuild her life but also inspired countless others along the way.

Today, Eunice is a powerful voice in the chronic illness community. She speaks openly about her journey with MS, challenging misconceptions about invisible disabilities and proving that it's possible to thrive—not just survive—while living with a chronic condition. Her philosophy of "Live. Don't claim it" has become a rallying cry for people facing various life challenges.

As a mother of three—including a son who keeps her active attending basketball games and two daughters pursuing their own dreams—Eunice demonstrates daily that having MS doesn't mean giving up on the things that matter most. She continues to be actively involved in her children's lives, showing them what resilience looks like in action.

Eunice uses mobility aids when needed, advocates for herself in medical settings, and has restructured her life to accommodate her condition while refusing to let it define her limitations. She cooks healthy meals at home, maintains an active social life with modifications that work for her, and has found new purpose in sharing her story with others.

Her upcoming speaking engagements at women's health programs represent her commitment to turning her pain into purpose, helping other women navigate their own health challenges with courage and hope. She believes strongly in the power of community, the importance of asking for help, and the possibility of finding joy and meaning even in the midst of difficult circumstances.

Through her advocacy work, Eunice addresses important issues including:

- The reality of living with invisible disabilities
- The importance of self-advocacy in healthcare settings
- The power of community support in healing

ABOUT THE AUTHOR

- The difference between surviving and thriving with chronic illness
- The role of faith and family in overcoming adversity

Eunice's story has already touched countless lives through personal conversations, community connections, and social media interactions. People regularly reach out to thank her for her openness about her MS journey and to share how her strength has inspired their own healing processes.

"The Day I Got Up" is Eunice's first book, but her impact as a voice of hope and resilience extends far beyond these pages. She continues to live in New York, where she remains deeply connected to her Harlem community while building bridges to support networks nationwide.

When she's not advocating for chronic illness awareness or spending time with her family, Eunice enjoys listening to music (which she considers medicine for the soul), cooking healthy meals at home, and finding creative ways to stay active within her physical capabilities.

Her message is simple but powerful: No matter what life throws at you, you have the strength to get back up. You are more than your circumstances. You deserve to live fully, love deeply, and never give up on the beautiful life that's still possible for you.

Eunice "Tweety" Newton proves every day that getting up isn't just possible—it's powerful.

For speaking engagements, interviews, or to connect with Eunice about her advocacy work, please contact 1Brick Publishing at info@1BrickPublishing.com

www.ingramcontent.com/pod-product-compliance
Lightning Source LLC
Chambersburg PA
CBHW070629030426
42337CB00020B/3957